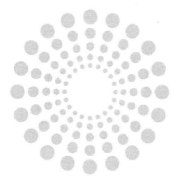

Thinfluence

Thinfluence

Thin-flu-ence (noun)
the powerful and surprising
effect friends, family,
work, and environment
have on weight

Walter Willett, MD, DRPH, Malissa Wood, MD,
Harvard Medical School, and Dan Childs

RODALE.

© 2014 by Harvard University

All rights reserved. No part of this publication may be reproduced or transmitted in any form or by any means, electronic or mechanical, including photocopying, recording, or any other information storage and retrieval system, without the written permission of the publisher.

Rodale books may be purchased for business or promotional use or for special sales. For information, please write to: Special Markets Department, Rodale Inc., 733 Third Avenue, New York, NY 10017.

Printed in the United States of America

Rodale Inc. makes every effort to use acid-free ⊗, recycled paper ♲.

The table on page 186 is reprinted from *Lancet,* Vol. 378, Boyd A. Swinburn et al, "The Global Obesity Pandemic," 801–14. Copyright 2011 with permission from Elsevier.

Book design by Jessica Morphew

Library of Congress Cataloging-in-Publication Data is on file with the publisher.
ISBN-13: 978-1-62336-015-3

Distributed to the trade by Macmillan
2   4   6   8   10   9   7   5   3   1   hardcover

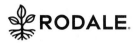

To our families

Contents

Introduction

You've dieted. You've exercised. And yet, you still find it a challenge to achieve a healthy weight and keep the extra pounds off.

How many times have you heard this story? Probably more than you can count. And you may have noticed that those around you are facing a similar struggle with their weight—your sister, your children, your co-workers, or your neighbors.

The ironic part is that, if this were any other problem that affected you and so many others you know—indeed, so many of the people living in this country—nearly all of us would immediately look to the underlying factors that contribute. During the most recent financial crisis, for example, individuals who were affected did not just scrutinize their own budgets and bank accounts; they looked at the home mortgage bubble, the practices by lending companies, and the policies of the federal government. Put another way, if the power goes out in a hurricane, you don't place all of the blame on your own fuse box. You're probably on the phone with the power company and looking out the window to see if your neighbors are experiencing the same issue.

The country finds itself in the midst of an obesity crisis, and so many other countries are already following suit. And yet, for most of us, when it comes to solving this problem, the approach we take is to "go it alone"—whether it involves a fad diet, an extreme exercise regimen, or some other narrowly focused strategy.

Clearly, the way we as individuals, as well as our society as a whole, should be engaging this problem is in a way that is completely opposite to the approach we have been taking. The personal lifestyle habits that we use to get to a healthier weight—and change it for good—should be supported within our families and homes. Our relationships outside of the home, too, should be more conducive to healthful choices and activities. Workplaces should be safe havens that foster health and healthy weight. And government entities should be responsive to the problem, enacting and enforcing policies that give all citizens, regardless of their socioeconomic background or geographical location, a better chance at being at a healthy weight.

Instead, unhealthy weight has been framed as an issue of individual responsibility, stigma, and personal shame. It is a portrayal that has seeped into the messages we get from the media and, hence, the myopic approaches that have been offered as solutions.

As Americans, most of us carry too much weight. Yet, there is little that is more isolating than trying to lose it.

What is the real solution? It is the thread that has the potential to connect all of the now disparate elements that contribute to our ability to achieve and maintain a healthy weight. This thread is influence—both the individual influence that we wield as well as the external influences that hold sway over what and how much we eat, the degree of physical activity we get, and the messages and policies that define the norms within our society.

Influence, of course, is a thread that connects many different areas that affect weight—nutrition and diet, exercise, relationships, and media messages to name just a few. So in order to appropriately tackle the issue and speak to all of these areas, I assembled a diverse team of authors to collaborate on this book.

My background is deeply rooted in food and agriculture. For five generations, the Willett family operated a dairy farm in Michigan, and I grew up actively involved in a 4-H vegetable club, taking home many blue ribbons at the local county fair and a state championship. I studied food science at Michigan State University before deciding to attend medical school to better understand the links between foods and health and to use this knowledge to help reduce the burden of illness. After obtaining my MD from the University of Michigan, I came to Harvard in Boston for internship and residency in internal medicine, still pursuing nutrition where possible along the way. Although I greatly enjoyed caring for my patients, I realized that most had conditions like heart disease and diabetes that could only be managed, not cured. Wanting to understand how these might, instead, be prevented, I enrolled in the doctoral program in epidemiology at Harvard School of Public Health. During this time, I began to develop ways to integrate the investigation of diet into long-term studies of risk factors for heart disease, cancer, and other important diseases. I applied these methods starting in 1980 in the Nurses' Health Study and the Health Professionals' Follow-Up Study. Together, these studies, which included nearly 300,000 men and women, provide the most detailed available information on the long-term health consequences of food choices.

Being a physician at heart, I realized that the many scientific papers we had published (more than 1,500!) needed to be shared in a way that could serve the general public. Thus, with the help of Ed Giovannucci and Pat Skerrett, I wrote *Eat, Drink, and Be Healthy: The Harvard Medical School Guide to Healthy Eating*, which documented the failure of the US Food Guide Pyramid to provide optimal guidance. In another book, *Eat, Drink, and Weigh Less*, I joined with Mollie Katzen to bring together the best available scientific evidence and culinary practices related to weight control. The scientific world has continued to identify powerful factors that influence our food choices both positively and negatively. *Thinfluence* offers this new knowledge in a way that can help you improve your own well-being and the lives of those around you.

In this book, I've partnered with two highly regarded experts. Dr. Malissa Wood is one of the leading preventive cardiologists in the United

States; she has led more than a dozen high-profile studies in the field. Her work also makes her an expert in the field of group approaches to healthy lifestyle changes. In her work as a clinical cardiologist, Dr. Wood frequently encounters patients who suffer from heart disease, and she is struck by the fact that in most cases, heart disease could have possibly been prevented. She decided early in her career that she could do more for her patients in the long run by teaching them how to make and stick with lifestyle changes rather than simply placing stents in the heart arteries and sending the patients on their way.

Dr. Wood has long observed the relationship between support from friends and family and success in weight loss in her patients. She works to help her patients change their behavior and encourages them to seek out the help of friends and family in supporting these changes. Dr. Wood also tries to lead by example and offers her patients suggestions for creating and maintaining an individual program of diet and exercise despite a busy schedule.

Trained at Harvard Medical School, Dr. Wood is currently codirector of the Corrigan Women's Heart Health Program at Massachusetts General Hospital (MGH). She is the lead investigator of the groundbreaking HAPPY Heart study at MGH, which educates participants on exercise, diet, and positive mental strategies to help them achieve happier, healthier lifestyles. Dr. Wood designed the HAPPY Heart study when she saw the benefits of combining health education with social supports in her practice but wanted to examine this relationship using scientific approach. She is a well-recognized champion for heart health whose involvement with the American Heart Association spans two decades. In 2009, Dr. Wood was recognized by the organization Best Doctors in America for her clinical and research excellence, and she serves as one of the cardiology experts on a multidisciplinary panel for this organization. Dr. Wood is a sought-after speaker and is able to articulate complex medical information to research scientists, physicians in clinical practice, and the public. She has been featured in many news articles and radio and television shows. She also speaks regularly at national cardiology meetings, sharing her research and wisdom with her colleagues and doctors in training.

Dan Childs is managing editor of the ABC News Medical Unit, the center of the news network's health and medical reporting. ABC News, among its various platforms, brings health and lifestyle information to hundreds of millions of Americans every month. Before heading the Medical Unit, Dan spent nearly a decade as a print medical journalist, writing hundreds of articles on topics including obesity, lifestyle, and health. Currently, he works with ABC News shows such as *Good Morning America* and *World News* in covering health and medical stories. But before this, as health editor for ABCNews.com, Dan saw the potential power of the Internet and social media in influencing decisions related to weight and health. He headed the OnCall+ resource center, an ABC News project that featured health and wellness videos in a Q&A format. Dan has been invited as a guest speaker at the Tufts Summer Institute on Digital Strategies for Health Communication as well as for the medical journalism program at the University of North Carolina at Chapel Hill, a program for which he is also a member of the advisory board. He also served as a panelist at the Association of Health Care Journalists (AHCJ) 2011 annual conference session on patient and health care consumer empowerment.

What we found as we explored the various factors that influence our health and risk of obesity was that there is no one, simple "magic bullet" solution to weight. Rather, there is an intricate interplay between many different elements in our day-to-day lives—some more obvious than others.

Understand this interplay, and it will become clear to you why your past weight-related resolutions have failed—and the things you can change to bring about real changes to your waistline and health that will stick. But more important, we will show you how to take steps that will spread to others, as well as the environment around you.

Are you ready to be a positive influence for weight change? It's time to get started!

—*Walter Willett, MD*

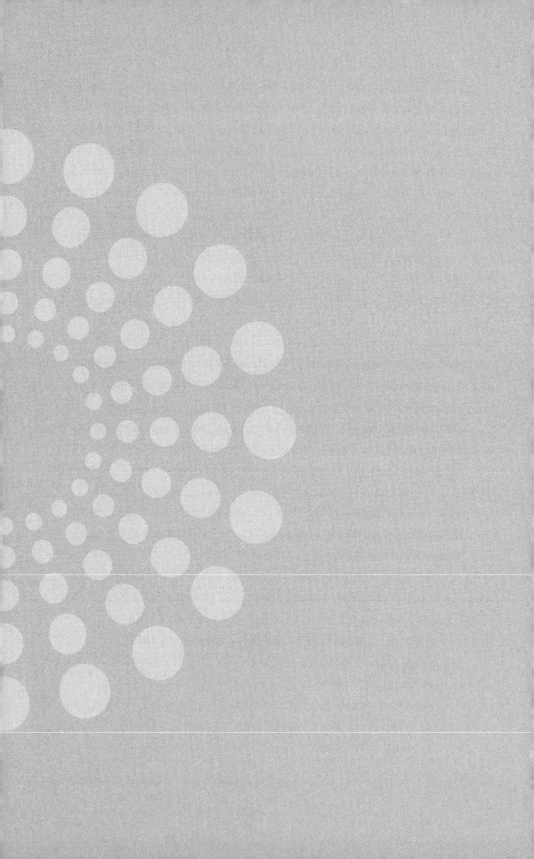

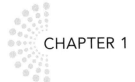

CHAPTER 1

What Is Thinfluence?

Young, thin, and healthy. Gabriela remembers this version of herself well from when she grew up in sunny Colombia, where she lived until she was thirty-three. Back then, she weighed 137 pounds. It may have been one of the last times she could remember being at a healthy weight for her five-foot, five-inch frame.

Indeed, many things were different when Gabriela lived in Colombia. When she recalls the tropical weather there, the balmy temperatures and the friendly layout of her community come to mind—the things that made her own two feet the ideal vehicle for getting from place to place. "I walked everywhere," she says, adding that she also owed some of her previous health to a good diet. "A lot of fruits, like pineapples, papaya, and vegetables. Everything was available at the market or from a cart."

Ultimately a job opportunity caused her to leave her home. And while the move would fulfill her dream of living in another country, she knew she'd have to make some adjustments. The climate was different, and so was the language. Feeling homesick, trying to make new friends—these changes were easy to anticipate. But alongside these expected challenges came alterations in her routine.

In Boston there were fewer opportunities for outdoor activities and exercise, particularly in winter. The fruits and vegetables with which she had been so familiar in Colombia and that had been a staple of her former diet were not as plentiful in Boston, and those that were available were more expensive. So, like the nearly imperceptible shifts in the New England seasons she now experienced, she gradually adopted a lifestyle that involved commuting instead of walking and pizza and fast food instead of fresh produce.

Not all of the adjustments were so difficult, and perhaps the most pleasant surprise Gabriela encountered was Rod. Unlike Gabriela, Rod had lived in the United States his entire life. He started smoking at an early age, but one day in 1997 he took his last drag on a cigarette and quit cold turkey. It was an important step for his health, and to this day Rod acknowledges kicking the smoking habit as a no-brainer. But for him, it was also the point at which his weight gain began.

"My average weight had been 152 pounds," he noted of his earlier years. "After I stopped smoking, I put on the weight and just kept eating."

It wouldn't seem like Rod and Gabriela would have much in common. But when she started working as a temp for his company in December 1999, they quickly grew close.

"It may have been love at first sight," he said with a laugh. "I can't remember. I just knew that I loved being around her."

Before long, their lives and their lifestyles had intertwined. For ten years they did everything together—shared meals, watched movies, spent time doing what they loved. And they also gradually gained weight together. By 2009, Rod tipped the scales at 242 pounds—officially obese. Gabriela weighed 158, which made her overweight for her height. Both were taking prescription medicines for high blood pressure and cholesterol by this time. Rod admitted that he showed up at the doctor's office "quite a bit" for chest pains, a very concerning sign.

"I did nothing," Rod recalls. "I just ate, lay on my bed looking at computers, and I stuffed my face with potato chips all day."

Like many couples in America today, both Rod and Gabriela needed a change. Indeed, their lives may have depended on it.

This change came first for Gabriela, after a particularly sobering checkup with her primary care physician. He referred her to the well-known HAPPY Heart program at Massachusetts General Hospital, which was designed to help women make healthy lifestyle changes. This is when she met Malissa, who headed the program. Looking back, Gabriela says the counseling and support she received through HAPPY Heart was the wake-up call that roused her from a routine that was slowly killing her.

It was not just a diet, nor was it simply an exercise program. It was a completely new kind of lifestyle. Gabriela began to eat more healthily. She started engaging in more physical activity. And after three years in the program, she was four pounds lighter—a modest amount of weight, but a difference nonetheless. And many of the positive effects were not ones that showed up on the scale. She lost fat and gained lean muscle mass, evidenced by the fact that her waist size dropped by more than four inches. Other measures of health, including her blood pressure and cholesterol, also improved. She found that she was able to cut back on some of her medications. Ask her today and she will tell you—emphatically—that she simply feels healthier.

But what about Rod? He joined no such program, and he didn't receive any special counseling or group support. And yet, for some reason, he, too, got better—much better.

In the same three years that Gabriela got lighter and healthier, Rod dropped a whopping seventy pounds. And in February 2012, he did something that just a few years might have seemed impossible to him and those who knew him well: He completed his first-ever 10-K race.

While all this was happening, another interesting transformation was occurring that, at first glance, would seem tangential at best to Rod's story. This transformation involved Rod's colleague, Larry, who happened to be in worse shape than Rod had been during his computer-and-potato-chip days. At his heaviest, Larry weighed almost four hundred pounds. These days, however, he is considerably lighter and can do something he has never been able to do before: He can join Rod on his regular jogs.

"Now that he's running with me," Rod says with a grin, "he looks like a different person."

These stories are separate and independent instances of three people's lives and lifestyles changing over the course of three years—or at least that is what our conventional views about weight loss would tell us. For years, the mantra of weight management has been one of self-discipline, of overcoming individual challenges. Sure, it is possible for us to view these changes in isolation. What would be the first thing you would say if these people were your friends or colleagues? It would likely be, "Wow, Larry looks so much better since he decided to make a change" or "Rod sure has taken it upon himself to improve his health."

Yet of these three people, Gabriela was the one whose healthy actions preceded those of the people connected to her in some way. So given that everyone lost weight in this story, we have two choices as to how to interpret exactly what happened. On the one hand, we could chalk it all up to happy coincidence. But while this is possible, it does not seem terribly likely. So on the other hand, we could venture that something else is going on here—that the actions of one person somehow influenced the actions of those she knew, and even those she did not know, for the better.

This "domino effect" of healthy behaviors has made headlines in recent years, almost always with a negative connotation. You might even remember some of them: "Your Friends Are Making You Fat," "Obesity Is Contagious, Study Finds," and "Can You Fight the Fat Flu?" among others. Many of these were spurred by the research of Nicholas Christakis, MD, PhD, of Harvard University and James Fowler, PhD, of the University of California, San Diego,[1] which found that if your sibling, spouse, or best friend is overweight, you are more likely to be overweight yourself. Specifically, the research showed that a person's chance of becoming obese increases by 57 percent if a close friend is obese, by 40 percent if a sibling is, and by 37 percent if their spouse is obese. This idea is broadly known as social contagion, and it goes a long way in explaining how habits, beliefs, and behaviors can spread throughout a group of connected individuals.

Perhaps the "contagion" part of this term makes us want to run away and wash our hands. It's not a word that we normally associate with good things. Yet follow-up research has shown us that it's not just negative health aspects that can be spread in this way. Take one 2011 study,[2] for instance, which found that individuals had greater intention to lose weight when one of their social contacts was trying to lose weight. Social contagion, it turns out, can be a vehicle for positive behaviors as well.

So for better or for worse, when scientists have examined how social connections relate to real-world outcomes like weight and obesity, they have found that the decisions we appear to make just for ourselves can ripple through the web of our social connections. They can influence those we know, and they can spread beyond our social circles, perhaps even beyond our communities, potentially influencing people to whom we may never be introduced.

Weight Loss: It's No Longer Just Personal

This clashes, of course, with much of what we've been conditioned to believe about our weight. It is no great leap to say that personal responsibility is perhaps the overriding theme in the arena of weight. On a daily basis, we hear an awful lot about our choices, our self-discipline, our need to slim down and get healthy. Even the most common phrases used to describe weight and weight loss usually lead us to believe that weight is an isolated, individual issue. Consider the following oft-heard statements:

◊ "I'm never going to lose these extra pounds."

◊ "She has put on so much weight."

◊ "Wow, did I ever let myself go!"

The truth is, however, that the notion that we are somehow islands when it comes to our weight simply isn't true. We have even begun to shift intuitively to understand this. Why else, for instance, would we be calling it an obesity "epidemic"? Think about it enough, and it soon becomes ironic that the issue of weight is so often framed as one in which we are "going it alone."

Not that anything is necessarily wrong with taking personal responsibility for adopting a healthier, more weight-friendly lifestyle. Few would argue that individual motivation and self-encouragement is a bad thing. Yet the language of personal responsibility when it comes to weight, all too often, is not at all encouraging. It is usually a language of blame. Being overweight has come to be viewed as a personal failure, a sign of weakness and vice. It is hardly the right foot to start from when devising broad strategies to solve the country's weight problem, and is far from constructive on the individual level, too.

Clearly it's time for a fresh start.

This fresh start is the principle behind *Thinfluence,* and the first step is realizing that the personal choices you make are enmeshed within a web of interconnected factors that reach far beyond simply what is on your plate or how long you spend on the treadmill. Once you recognize these various factors as what they are, you will be able to turn them in your favor. This is what sets *Thinfluence* apart from everything you think you know about the reasons you have put on weight, why your past efforts to lose weight have failed, and how you can move forward with real, sustainable strategies to improve.

Your Weight Is Not Your Fault

You have probably heard the following mathematical equation many times in the past: Calories consumed minus calories expended equals the deficit that you need to achieve your weight goals. Technically speaking, this is absolutely true—if you burn more than you take in, you will lose weight, and if you burn less than you take in, you will gain it. It's simple math.

The problem is this: Few, if any, of us live our lives like a mathematical equation. While certain situations may make it easy for us to count calories in and calories out, this strategy becomes much harder to follow during holiday visits to the in-laws, where second helpings at the Thanksgiving table are *de rigueur,* or when a late evening at the office means skipping the gym and going in with your colleagues on delivery pizza.

Other factors beyond diet and exercise make it more difficult for us to exert control over our weight. Start by taking a look at the elements of your environment. Consider your kitchen pantry or fridge. When you open either of them, are you presented with healthy yet satisfying options for meals and snacks? Or are you more likely to find bottles of sugary soda staring back at you? Notice how close your television is to the area where you eat your meals. Is it positioned in a way that fosters TV watching while you eat, a distraction that can lead you to eat more than you intended? Look out your living room window. Do you see a sidewalk? A busy thoroughfare? How far is it to the nearest grocery store? The answers to these questions may be more impactful to your weight and health than you realize.

Many other things that hold sway over your weight may be even more surprising. These could include your paycheck, the politics of your local and national government, and other seemingly external factors. And there is science to prove it. For example, in a landmark study published in the *New England Journal of Medicine*,[3] researchers demonstrated for the first time that simply moving out of a neighborhood with a high level of poverty into one with a lower level of poverty was linked to a 13 percent reduction in the risk of moderate-risk obesity—in other words, having a body mass index greater than 35.

We encounter influences like these and more every day. They are often so commonplace and subtle, they have become invisible—until they hit our waistlines, that is. These "blind spots" affect our efforts to lose or maintain our weight. And their impact is considerable.

The good news is this: By realizing that these spots exist, you are halfway toward bending them in your favor. Think about it—what would you be able to achieve in terms of your weight, your appearance, and your health if your family and close friends reinforced what you were doing? Or if your workplace became conducive to exercise? Or if you were routinely able to cut calories from your diet before entering the grocery store checkout line?

These approaches may not come to your mind first in terms of improving your weight. But they are vital to consider, and they're exactly the types of things we will be discussing in the chapters to come.

Can You Be an Influence for Weight Change?

As we discuss these oft-overlooked factors that impact weight, it may have already occurred to you that many of them are the very things that link us to the people we work with, know, and love. What this tells us is clear: Not only are we on the receiving end of the influence, but we, too, can have a positive effect on those around us.

As it turns out, this is precisely what happened for Gabriela and Rod. What we know about the spread of healthy behaviors through a social network strongly suggests that Rod caught a healthy "bug" from his wife, which he in turn passed on to his friend Larry at work. When Gabriela began to eat differently and exercise more, Rod says that he began, almost unconsciously, to make changes that helped him avoid "stuffing his face." As unhealthy foods began disappearing from the cupboards and the dinner table, a healthier lifestyle became the path of least resistance. "She would say stuff to me as well, like, 'Get some exercise! Do something!'" he recalls.

Inspired by his wife, Rod began going to the gym every night. Instead of heavy, calorie-laden lunches, he'd bring fruit and other healthy options to work. In the evenings, salads began to replace steaks. Before long, Larry noticed the changes in Rod, which inspired him to start exercising himself. Whether it was a yearning for camaraderie or the pangs of a healthy competitive spirit, Larry worked out on his own until he was fit enough to join Rod on his regular jogs. And it's likely that Larry's behavior change had an effect on his family, his neighbors, and the members of his church. Then as those people adopted healthier habits, they had an impact on other people in their lives. When you think of it this way, Gabriela's resolution to adopt a healthier lifestyle not only changed the numbers she saw on her scale, but affected the lifestyle and weight of countless others as well—both those who were closely connected to her and people with whom she had little, if any, contact.

Indeed, it is likely that if we had the power to see Gabriela's social network as a flowchart, we would see her reach extend in many directions other than the chain that began with Rod. It's likely when she talked to her family in Colombia, they recognized what a positive change her new routine made in her life, which perhaps gave them incentive to make healthy changes as well. Or she very well may have inspired her work friends in some way, small or large, to adopt healthier lifestyle habits and achieve a healthier weight. Whatever the effect, it is safe to say that Gabriela's resolution to live a healthier life reached far beyond her own personal experience.

Your Circles of Influence

Admittedly, we've given you quite a bit to digest here. We've told you that the concerns you have about your weight not only may have to do with what you are putting in your mouth or how often you hit the treadmill at the gym, but could be directly related to what your friends are doing, what your office looks like, and even the decisions made by your town council. It is a lot to consider, especially since some of these aspects may be more out of your direct control than others.

For you to come up with strategies to improve your situation, it is crucial that you have an easy way to visualize the things that are influencing your decisions and actions. This is where the "Circles of Influence" come in.

Each chapter of *Thinfluence* covers a different category of influences that we confront daily—from our own internal issues to those within our social networks, all the way to broad, societal influences. Take a look at the illustration on page 10. This graph represents all of the various influences, from individual to global, that have an impact on your health, your weight, and the decisions you make every day.

This model places you, the individual, in the middle of the figure. Your family connections reside in the next circle, and in the next one are your social influences, including your friends and work colleagues.

The next circle contains environmental influences, such as your physical environment and what we term your food environment. The outer circle represents broad, societal factors such as government policies and global economic forces.

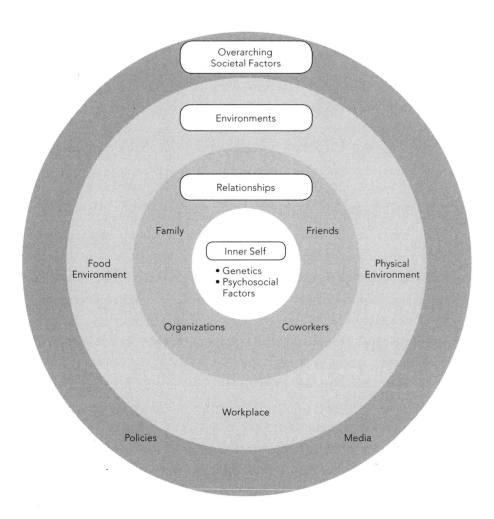

The principles that govern this graph are simple:

◊ The inner circles represent areas over which you have the most direct control.

◊ The factors in the inner circles have the most direct impact on your weight and health.

◊ The farther out a circle is from the center, the less direct control you have over the factors it contains.

◊ The factors in the outermost circles have the least direct impact on your weight and health, but they still likely play an important role.

No memorization of this basic road map is necessary at this point. All you need to know for now is that you wield a certain amount of influence in the various areas of your life, and while making changes in some of these areas might be easier than in others, you do have the power to turn the tables on the factors in your life that are leading to an unhealthy weight.

In other words, there is a practical side to the current research on social and environmental factors and our weight, and we are going to show you how to take full advantage of these findings to conquer your own weight battle.

But here's the really cool part. As you may have gathered from this discussion of the power of various influences affecting your weight, influence is a two-way street.

In fact, just for fun, let's think about what would happen if you inspired others through your own healthy changes to make healthy changes as well. What if those you inspired, in turn, inspired others? In its loftiest form, a bending of the curve on unhealthy weight in this country could follow. You have taken a positive step in picking up this book, not just for yourself, but potentially for countless others whom you will never meet. They all have a stake—and society in general has a stake—in your health and weight. It seems incredible, and yet this is really the central message of our book.

Through the following pages, our goal together will be simple: to help you find the tools and strategies you need to become a force for positive lifestyle change not just in your own life, but in the lives of those you know and love, and in turn the ones they know and love. You will gain a greater understanding of how aspects of our social connections and the environment in which we live affect our weight and health, and we will show you how to use this knowledge to your advantage. You'll learn how to identify the positive and negative influences in your life and how to avoid, circumvent, or change them. Moreover, once you understand the social and environmental influences that lead to weight gain, you will be able to spread your own positive influence through your social networks and physical environment—leading your family, your friends, and your co-workers to a healthier weight as well.

Are you ready to get started? Good! Let's begin with your plan of action.

Thinfluence Action Plan

As you progress through this book, we hope you will find that *Thinfluence* is not a prefabricated, one-size-fits-all set of recommendations for everyone who reads it. Rather it is a guide that will help you formulate your own plans and solutions to achieve the results you desire.

The framework we will carry through every chapter in this book consists of three parts:

◊ Analyze

◊ Act

◊ Influence

That's it. A convenient three-step process in every chapter—a one-two-three punch that will help you make the most of what you learn from looking at the factors in your life that powerfully influence your weight.

The first step is Analyze. In this step, we will help you explore various areas of your life through a quick questionnaire. More than just a simple Q-and-A, it is designed to help you take note of the hidden factors that may be helping or hindering your efforts to change or control your weight.

In the Act step, we will help you interpret the meaning behind your answers. This is also the part where you will develop your personal toolbox from suggestions we provide, depending on your situation and needs. Everyone will need to use a different set of tools. The important thing is that the solutions you end up with will address the challenges you are facing and are within your power to execute.

The final step, Influence, is the realization of the success of your chosen solutions. In essence, we want you to look forward to the desired impact of your actions. This step will allow you to take some time to consider the impact you will have, which will arm you with convincing incentives to make these changes. While this is important to keep yourself motivated, it is also the basis for your ability to convince others to make these positive changes as well. You will be not only strengthening your own resolve, but building teams that will both help your teammates and support you in your efforts.

Taken together, these three steps will help you build what we refer to as your Thinfluence Action Plan, which will serve as a guide for you going forward. As for how you choose to record and update this plan, it's fine to use an old-fashioned notebook or the latest technological device—whichever is the most comfortable for you. We hope that your action plan will be a guide you can refer to over and over again, long after you finish reading this book.

Below we will walk through an example of what these steps could be for a person reading this book. You will, of course, have your own situation to which you can apply this one-two-three approach. But perhaps the "dry run" below will give you a taste of the steps through which we will be guiding you.

Thinfluence Action Plan: Laying It All Out

If you were cooking a meal, it's fair to say that the best way to start would be to lay out all of the ingredients where you could see them. This is a bit like how the Thinfluence Action Plan works—except that instead of laying out the ingredients that make up a meal, you'll want to take stock of the ingredients of your life that are likely to be affecting your weight.

ANALYZE

1. How do you feel about the choices those around you are making that relate to their weight?

A. Terrible! The people I spend time with tend toward unhealthy diet choices and are mostly sedentary.

B. So-so. While some people I spend time with have healthy lifestyle habits, there are others whose definition of "living it up" almost always involves overindulging.

C. Great! Most if not all of those I spend time with practice healthy lifestyle habits—and they seem to have fun as well.

2. When you consider the physical environments where you live and work, the word most likely to come to mind is:

A. Toxic. My home and workplace are not set up for physical activity, and junk food is never far from reach.

B. Neutral. It may not be the most encouraging environment for physical activity, but exercise is at least a possibility. And there is always a choice between healthy and less-healthy food options.

C. Healthy! My environment is geared toward physical activity and healthy eating.

3. Think about your neighborhood and community. What kind of priority is placed on healthy living?

A. Low. Rarely, if ever, do I hear about healthy initiatives being implemented in the place where I live, nor have I come across any groups within my community that are trying to change this picture.

B. Medium. A few groups and organizations within the community are pushing for healthier behaviors, and the community is home to at least some efforts to improve the health of its inhabitants.

C. High. From walking trails to community events, the place where I live screams healthy!

ACT

In this section, we will look at your answers and help with strategies to accentuate the positive influences and counteract the negatives.

◊ Mostly As: Don't despair. While this is a challenging starting point, many people find themselves in the same situation. This may even be one of the reasons you picked up this book. So if you currently are in an unhealthy situation, you are in the right frame of mind to start making changes—even simple ones—that have real potential to help you achieve your weight goals and possibly be a positive influence for others in your life.

◊ Mostly Bs: You're actually starting from a pretty good place, all things considered. This doesn't mean that the factors in your life are perfectly aligned to help you with your weight. But it does mean that resources are around you in the form of healthy friends, living situations that are amenable to exercise, and community resources. Find these resources and use them to their full extent.

◊ Mostly Cs: Congratulations! It seems that you have an excellent starting point, both socially and environmentally, to improve your weight. Your goal should be to take full advantage of the gifts that surround you.

Meanwhile, here are some of the things you can do right now to act on this information, no matter what situation you are in:

◊ Make a short list of the three things you feel influence your diet and exercise choices the most. This could be a good friend, a living situation, a routine, or something else.

◊ Referring to the three things you just jotted down, write down one or two things you feel you could do differently in order to live a bit healthier. These will be the first areas for you to consider when making positive changes, however small.

INFLUENCE

Once you have your list of solutions, come up with some "selling points" you can use both to keep yourself motivated and to encourage others to join you in your plan to achieve a healthier weight. Here's what this might look like:

Goal: Healthier behaviors among your family, friends, and other social groups

Incentive: An improved sense of camaraderie in working toward a healthy end, not to mention a healthier weight for you

Goal: Achieving a home and working environment that is more conducive to activities leading to a healthier weight

Incentive: Improving your odds of putting healthy resolutions into practice, no matter where you are

Goal: Being part of community efforts that encourage weight-healthy lifestyles

Your Thinfluence Toolbox

A toolbox is a selection of options and tactics from which you can choose to give yourself a customized plan to accomplish your goals. At the end of each chapter, in the "Act" portion of the Thinfluence Action Plan, we will offer you ways to add to your toolbox. Here are some helpful tips to get the most out of this strategy:

◊ Find what works for you. The best options will be the ones that fit your goals, preferences, and lifestyle—not necessarily the ones that work for everyone else.

◊ Set goals for yourself. This is tremendously important. Even simple lifestyle changes are not always easy, and having a concrete goal will give you motivation to press on.

◊ Start small. Even if you pick just one small thing to do today, that could be the nudge you need to get going. And it could pave the way for bigger changes.

Incentive: A healthier environment not just for you, but for the rest of your town or neighborhood as well

With these incentives in hand, you will be coming to your social group armed with the reasons they should join you and support you in your efforts. All the more important, then, to record all of your observations in your Thinfluence Action Plan.

So after this first exercise, you should have written down or otherwise recorded a short list of actionable strategies you can put into motion immediately. And as you progress through the following chapters, you will be able to design more and more of these individually tailored strategies to incorporate into your day-to-day life.

Fighting the Inertia of Your Current Routine

By reading this far—even if you haven't started your Thinfluence Action Plan—you have already taken the first step on a journey that will give you a better understanding of what is affecting your weight and health, as well as the steps you can take to change these factors.

At first it might seem like a tough climb. It is important to bear in mind that not all of the strategies you come up with will be simple enough to put into motion. Habit is a very powerful force, and some routines will take a great deal of work to change, particularly since they may involve people you love and spend a great deal of time with.

The important thing to remember is that starting simple—doing even one good thing—may lead to real results. More important, a small change right away could serve as a stepping-stone to bigger, more impactful changes later on.

So as you progress through this book and identify the factors that influence your weight and health, realize that applying what you learn does not mean you will need to take drastic actions, like shuffling your friends-and-family deck, changing your job, or moving to another state. What it does mean is that you will become aware of the ways that the people and other forces in your life are contributing to your weight—and in turn, how your actions and influence may be contributing to theirs.

These back-and-forth influences form the basis for the idea of *Thinfluence*. But before you can understand these interactions and apply what you will be learning to your life, you first need to become more aware of what you bring to this equation—in other words, the individual qualities that determine how you influence others and how you let yourself be influenced. In the next chapter, we will take an introspective look at the genetic, psychological, social, and other factors that affect your weight, as well as the weight of those around you. And what you find out may surprise you.

What Is a Social Network Anyway?

When we use the term *social network*, it may be tempting to think about popular social media applications such as Facebook and Twitter. But in reality, your social network is much larger than this, and you don't even need to use a computer to have one.

You can think of your social network as everyone you know and interact with, plus everyone they know and interact with, and so on. The people you personally know and interact with each day are in your first-degree social network. Your second-degree network consists of the people known by those in your first-degree network, but not by you, and so on.

As an example, let's say that you have a sister. She has a husband, and he has a best friend. That best friend of your sister's husband would be three degrees of separation from you. If that best friend had a wife, that would be four degrees, and so on.

What Is a Healthy Diet?

Almost everyone agrees that eating a healthy diet is good, but when defining what a healthy diet is, opinions often diverge: very low fat, high protein, very low carbohydrate, MyPyramid, and many more. Fortunately, the last decades of research have given us a much better understanding of dietary characteristics that promote long-term health and well-being, and the good news is that there are many ways to have a healthy diet. The critical features are:

◊ Healthy fats, which include almost all vegetable oils such as olive oil, soybean oil, and corn oil (trans fat should be avoided and animal fats kept low)

◊ Healthy forms of carbohydrates, mainly high-fiber, whole grains

◊ Healthy forms of protein, meaning little or no red meat, and emphasis on vegetable protein sources such as nuts and beans with modest amounts of fish, poultry, eggs, and dairy products

◊ Abundant intake of vegetables (potatoes don't count) and fruits (easy on bananas, and little or no fruit juice)

◊ Minimal or no sugar-sweetened beverages, but water, coffee, and tea are great (alcohol in moderation if consumed)

We don't mention any specific percentages of fat, sugar, or carbohydrate because much research shows that it is not critical to do so if all are healthy versions of these "macronutrients." This allows great potential for variety and individual preferences.

Of the traditional dietary patterns, the Mediterranean diet best fits the definition of a healthy diet, emphasizing fruits and vegetables, whole grains, fish, nuts, and healthy fats like olive oil. Understanding these elements allows us to create healthy eating patterns with flavors and traditions from all over the world. Most important, a healthy diet must provide enjoyment and flexibility so it can be sustained for a lifetime. We are not talking about a crash diet that leads to temporary weight loss and then failure.

If you want more details about healthy eating, read the scientific evidence in a book for a general audience, *Eat, Drink, and Be Healthy: The Harvard Medical School Guide to Healthy Eating.*

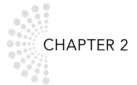

CHAPTER 2

Know Thyself: Internal Factors That Affect Your Weight . . . and How External Factors Influence Them

When it comes to your weight, is it all on you?

As we discussed earlier, one of the biggest misconceptions about weight control is that it is a wholly individual issue. For this reason, many approaches to weight loss and weight control—including most fad diets— stop at the self when making positive changes. The implication is clear: You are solely responsible for where you are with your weight. And what happens with your weight from here on out is simply a product of your personal traits. Among the most common traits you may blame for your weight are:

◊ Your genes

◊ Your emotions and feelings

◊ Your "addiction" to food

We hear about these three factors a lot. And almost always, they are presented as things we are responsible for ourselves, even if we can't always control them directly.

This, of course, can lead to a very lonely and isolating road to change. Stumble along the path, and the failed effort starts to look like a personal failure. In light of this, it's little wonder that weight issues can carry with them such a stigma!

Clearly internal factors matter, and all of us face them in one form or another. Those internal factors can hold sway over our power to make healthy choices—our ability to motivate ourselves, our mindfulness of our behaviors, and our resolve to stay the course once we have made a change.

But while most of us are aware of the effect that inner factors have on our weight, more often than not we tend to think about them in the wrong way—a way that ends with us blaming ourselves unreasonably.

The truth is that many of these internal factors are influenced and shaped more by external factors than most people realize.

So if a single concept in this book is important to understand, it is that many of the things we traditionally view as "our own problem" in terms of our weight—things like our genes, our emotions, and even our chances of being addicted to food—are actually very much linked to forces outside of ourselves.

Bear in mind, too, that this is not a one-way street. We can harness and adapt aspects of our behaviors and choices to encourage a healthier dynamic in other areas of our lives.

What Inner Factors Can Mean for Your Weight

How much impact can inner factors have on what we weigh? In her work to promote wellness by improving diets and lifestyle factors, Malissa has helped many individuals who have struggled with inner factors that affect their weight. Some themes occur repeatedly.

Take, for example, a woman we will refer to as Amelia. She was thin in childhood and adolescence, but after the birth of her children, her relationship with food took a turn for the worse. The stress of managing her home, her job, and her relationships took a toll on Amelia. When faced with difficulty, she turned to the one friend who never was too busy or preoccupied to spend time with her—food. The busier her life became, the more Amelia turned to her new best friend, and she quickly piled on the weight. Amelia saw her body mass index (BMI) creep from the "overweight" to "obese" range. Before she knew it, she had gained fifty pounds and developed medical complications of obesity: prediabetes, high blood pressure, and arthritis in her knees. As her waistline grew, her self-confidence plummeted and her marriage started to crumble. Only when faced with the loss of her health and her husband did she seek counseling. Fortunately, she came to recognize the cycle of dependence on food as a crutch to deal with stress and developed other coping mechanisms. Malissa now monitors Amelia from time to time for mild high blood pressure, but she has lost fifty pounds through diet and increased exercise.

Another woman, Beth, is morbidly obese. She has been able to exercise, but she just can't seem to stay away from food and wine. They have become her passion. Beth has told Malissa that indulging in this way is really all she looks forward to at this point in her life. She is single, works as a paralegal, and is lonely. Each day, she retreats to her home, where she greets her best friends—food and wine. Despite the fact that multiple health complications now limit her activities, she has no interest in losing weight at this point.

Two different stories, but one thing in common: Both illustrate the challenge many people face from inner factors—both physical and psychological—that play an important role in their weight problems. They also demonstrate how closely intertwined these inner factors can become with external factors, such as our relationships and day-to-day routines.

So as we embark on this journey to better understand the universe of influences that affect your weight, let's use these inner factors as a starting point.

Getting to Know Your "Inner-Self" Factors

When you think about how your inner-self factors relate to the external factors that affect your weight, it might be useful to imagine yourself navigating a sailboat on the open sea. Even if you have no nautical experience, it is easy to imagine how you would have to move the rudder and trim the sails to get where you want to be. These are the things inside the boat—the inner factors—over which you have the most direct control. The direction of the wind, the choppiness of the water, or the approaching storm front are the external factors largely outside of your control. Yet for a skillful navigator who understands the tricks of the sport, it is often possible to circumvent the outside influences that threaten to steer the boat off its course and perhaps even use these influences to his or her advantage.

What, specifically, do we mean when we talk about these inner factors? While there are perhaps too many to discuss in this chapter alone, many of them fit into one of the three important categories that we mentioned on page 21.

Inner-Self Factor #1: Genetics

Perhaps the "innermost" inner factor behind your weight is what you inherit from your parents. We've long known that a propensity toward being overweight can "run in the family," a fact that you might be reminded of every time you have a family reunion. But recently researchers have learned even more about the specific genes that influence our weight.

For years researchers have been aware of certain genetic variations that increase an individual's chances of being overweight. These variations were thought to be rare but in 2007 scientists managed to tease out the first common genetic contributor to obesity,[1] a gene they christened "fat mass and obesity associated gene." Hardly an imaginative label, but it was descriptive at least. The official symbol of this gene was designated FTO, and you may recognize this moniker from news stories on the topic.

Everyone has the FTO gene. What matters is that we can have many variations of this gene. In other words, your FTO gene may not be exactly the same as somebody else's. Moreover, scientists have linked several variations of this gene to greater daily intake of calories and, consequently, a higher risk of overweight or obesity.

Since the initial findings on the FTO gene, researchers have uncovered dozens of other "fat genes" that are each associated with a slightly increased risk of overweight or obesity. If we have the "fatter" version of most of these genes, which is quite uncommon, our risk of obesity is approximately doubled compared to someone with the "thinner" version of all these genes.

These gene variations are common: It is thought that nearly two-thirds of people of European or African descent carry a version of a gene that puts them at greater risk of being overweight or obese, and nearly half of Asians do. And for some the effects of these genes carry more impact than for others. Say, for example, that both of your parents carry the "fatter" version of the FTO gene and pass it on to you. This would mean that your risk of being overweight or obese would be higher—almost twice as high, in this case—than that of someone who did not get this version of the FTO gene from either parent.

Finding genes that are tied to our weight is important and potentially useful. With further study, researchers may be able to use this knowledge to better understand obesity and possibly even devise new treatments for those who need them.

When these findings were picked up by the news media, the flurry of coverage that followed solidified a potentially discouraging notion: that we are all born with a certain weight destiny. Consider the following headlines that ran shortly after the findings on FTO came to light:

◊ Like Fatty Foods? Blame Your Genes

◊ Are You Obese? Blame It on Your Genes

◊ We've Found the Gene That Makes You Fat, Claim Scientists Studying Obesity

The message was clear: Have the right gene and you have a chance of losing weight. Have the wrong one and get ready for an uphill battle. It was a disheartening philosophy and also, for the most part, an unfortunate misinterpretation of perfectly legitimate and important genetic research.

Setting the record straight was a large review study published in 2011 in the journal *PLoS Medicine* by an international team of researchers.[2] The researchers crunched the data from forty-five studies to see what the real impact of the FTO gene was with regard to weight status in adults.

What they found was actually encouraging: Adults bequeathed with the "fat" gene by their parents were not condemned to a life of obesity. Those with the gene did indeed have a higher chance of being heavier, but regular physical activity cut the effect of this gene on obesity by about a third. Moreover, the researchers found that having one copy of the gene appeared to be responsible for, on average, only about two extra pounds of excess weight. Not fifty pounds, not even twenty. Two pounds. All thirty-two ounces of which can potentially be countered with the right lifestyle changes. Even having two copies of this version of the FTO gene, one from each parent, is associated with only about seven extra pounds on average.

In fact, in many cases, these gene variations may only "kick in" once they are triggered by other lifestyle factors.

One study that supports this idea was published in the journal *Circulation*.[3] Lu Qi, MD, PhD; Walter; and colleagues at Harvard found that among those who had genetic variations linked to being overweight, a sedentary lifestyle—in this case defined as watching more than forty hours of TV each week—appeared to be the trigger for weight gain. The effects of the fat genes in these subjects were about four times greater than the effects seen in others who had these same genetic variations but who spent less than an hour per week watching TV. Moreover, those who had such a genetic predisposition but instead used their leisure time to engage in physical activity equivalent to an hour per day of brisk walking cut the effect of their fat genes nearly in half.

It's not just our level of physical activity that can determine whether these genes kick in or not. In another study published in the *New England Journal of Medicine*,[4] a team composed of many of the same researchers, including Walter, examined a similar connection in those who had a genetic variant associated with obesity and their consumption of sugary beverages. They found that the more servings per week of sugar-sweetened beverages that an individual with the fat gene variations reported, the more of an effect these genes appeared to have on their weight. So again, the research reveals that while these genes raise the risk of gaining weight, it is the lifestyle-related risk factor of high-calorie beverage consumption that "springs the trap," leading to weight gain.

So for most people, the factors that tip the scales toward weight gain are things we can control. This is a very hopeful message. It means you may have more potential for control over your weight than you might have guessed. And this realization alone may be a significant step toward a healthy change.

Once we take to heart the findings of these studies, it should be clear that even in the face of gene variations that influence our weight, the real power lies in our own hands. This may go a long way in explaining why weight problems are so prevalent in the United States. Despite the prevalence of these gene variations worldwide, you would be hard-pressed to find a country in which a significant percentage of the population does not have them. The bottom line, in other words, is that genetics cannot explain the obesity epidemic. The explosion of weight problems that Americans now face is a relatively recent phenomenon, one that has come about too quickly to blame genetic change, which happens very slowly. More important, we know that Americans are genetically similar to other people living in countries from which their ancestors emigrated—yet obesity rates vary largely across countries. For example, in Japan and Sweden the obesity rates are about 5 percent in women, but in the United States the rates are almost 40 percent. Interestingly, when women relocate from Sweden or Japan to the United States, research shows that they tend to fatten up and look much more like Americans.[5,6]

If it were all up to these genes alone, rates of overweight and obesity would be roughly the same everywhere. And we know they are not.

Inner-Self Factor #2: Emotions

In a perfect world, all of us would eat for one reason and one reason alone: because we are hungry. However, anyone who has ever spent a boring day in front of the TV . . . or has reached into the freezer for the ice cream when a relationship has gone sour . . . or has stayed up late into the night working on a stressful project . . . will know firsthand that this is not the case.

Our feelings and emotions at any particular time have a very real effect on our choices of when and what to eat. And while external factors have a big effect on how we are feeling—the status of our relationship or the demands of our job, for example—our emotions should be considered an inner factor behind our weight for some very good reasons.

For one, the way we process our experience into an emotion is unique to each of us. We may not always feel as if we are in complete control of how situations or events impact our emotional state, but the fact remains that this is an internal process.

Secondly, psychological conditions—like depression and anxiety—can hold sway over our emotions. Those who experience these know that they can influence many of the choices made and the actions taken on a day-to-day basis. And many of these choices and actions, in turn, have an effect on weight.

Depression's role in weight status is especially interesting, since recent research suggests that depression and weight may be more closely intertwined than most of us realize. One of these studies[7] analyzed data from the famous Nurses' Health Study, one of the longest-running and most extensive investigations ever conducted of the various factors that influence

What BMI Means . . . And What It Really Means for You

When we talk about a healthy weight, what does it really mean? The measure you have probably seen most is the one we described earlier as body mass index or BMI, and it is calculated using the following formula:

$$BMI = \text{Your weight in kilograms} / (\text{height in meters})^2$$

Most health experts currently consider this measure the gold standard, but that does not mean it is the best indicator for everyone. Take, for example, a superhealthy bodybuilder who has a great deal of muscle mass for his height; in this example, a high BMI would not be an indicator of obesity. On the other hand, for many people a BMI of 23 or 24 is too high, even though it is not conventionally considered an indication that someone is overweight.

One measure other than BMI that may be helpful is waist circumference, since accumulation of fat around the abdomen is strongly linked with such problems as coronary artery disease, stroke, and type 2 diabetes—even when BMI is taken into account. In the United States, health experts often consider a waist circumference of one hundred centimeters for men and eighty-eight centimeters for women to be the upper "healthy" limit. True, for some people this limit would be far higher than desirable. But researchers have suggested that monitoring changes in waist circumference might be a useful way to determine whether lifestyle interventions are necessary.[8] For example, if an individual has added five centimeters to his or her waist in a given time period, a health care professional might use that as a basis for determining that changes in activity patterns and diet are needed.

women's health. Walter has been a lead investigator on the study since its inception in 1976. At this time, researchers began the project that would eventually gather volumes of information on the health and behaviors of more than 200,000 women, and since then they have been comparing these factors against each other to tease out the relationships between them. In one such analysis, An Pan, PhD, formerly of the Harvard School of Public Health's department of nutrition led a team that investigated the relationship between depression status and the risk of being obese in middle-age women. They determined that women who were depressed at the beginning of the study period were 38 percent more likely to be obese by the end of the study. But they also found that, likewise, the women who were obese at the beginning of the study were 11 percent more likely to be depressed at the end of the study than their normal-weight counterparts. In other words, Dr. Pan and his colleagues showed what health experts call a bidirectional relationship: These factors appear to operate in both directions. In light of this, one can imagine a vicious cycle of unhealthy weight and depression, with one of these factors increasing the likelihood of the other and vice versa.

Depression, of course, is only one example of an emotional condition that is linked to our weight. Stress, boredom, or a simple case of the blues may be all it takes for some of us to make less-than-healthy choices in what we eat and how much activity we get. For some of us, a lonely evening with nothing to do is the trigger to search the fridge. For others, a bout of anxiety in the face of an important deadline can knock us out of our gym routine. And many can attest that the end of a relationship may be all it takes to make us reach for a pint of Ben & Jerry's.

The way our emotional state influences our food choices is particularly interesting. Science even tells us that there's a good reason why we call some tasty and often high-calorie treats "comfort food:" What we eat can often take our minds off our troubles and stressors, at least temporarily. The effects of indulging in comfort foods do not live only in our stomachs; they live in our heads as well. This is what researchers at the University of Cincinnati College of Medicine found when investigating how comfort foods work.[9] Specifically, they saw that engaging in what they called "palatable snacking"—think gobbling down a stack of Oreos with a glass of chocolate milk—may actually dampen the nervous system's response to stress. Their conclusion? "Stress tends to alter the pattern of

Is Emotional Eating an Issue for You?

While you may hear a lot about emotional eating, it might be hard to tell whether you do it or not. The three questions below are adapted from a commonly used assessment known as the Three-Factor Eating Questionnaire.[10]

1. When I feel anxious, I find myself eating.

   Definitely true (4)
   Mostly true (3)
   Mostly false (2)
   Definitely false (1)

2. When I feel blue, I often overeat.

   Definitely true (4)
   Mostly true (3)
   Mostly false (2)
   Definitely false (1)

3. When I feel lonely, I console myself by eating.

   Definitely true (4)
   Mostly true (3)
   Mostly false (2)
   Definitely false (1)

Take a look at your answers to these questions. Without even tallying up your score, you might realize from your responses that you are eating emotionally more than you initially thought. If your total score on these questions is 10 or above, you may want to talk to your doctor about the possibility that you are engaging in emotional eating. He or she will be able to discuss with you the next steps you can take to break the emotional eating cycle.

Remember: This is nothing to feel bad or ashamed about, as emotional eating affects many, many people. The important thing is recognizing the problem.

food consumption, and promotes craving of [calorie]-dense comfort foods."

In other words—let's face it—many of us live with an internal struggle between our dietary id and ego. Sometimes when our lives and stress levels leave us feeling "tapped out," we seek to feed the id. In an effort to replenish our energy and appetite, we relinquish control and look away from the downside of thoughtless eating. Our id is happy, but we eventually wake up to our ego—and the scales. Our dietary id can cunningly convince us we need "comfort food," while in actuality it should be called "discomfort food"—because trying to squeeze a size 12 body into size 8 jeans is anything but comfortable!

But it's not just stress. We are finding more evidence of a biological component to eating that results from such emotions as anxiety or even just plain boredom. Because these are emotional responses that come up so often in our day-to-day lives—whether we're talking about interpersonal stress at home or among our friends, or work-related stress when scrambling to complete an important project—the eating patterns that result from them can cause us to sabotage our best weight-control efforts in a dangerously surreptitious way.

The most important step in breaking the cycle of emotional eating is recognizing when it is happening. And the key to this is a concept known as mindfulness. When you reach for comfort foods in times of emotional stress, do you know you are doing it?

The good news is that a bit of mindfulness can go a long way toward recognizing and correcting these behavior patterns. More often than not, it simply involves paying attention to our actions in the face of a stressful situation. Kelly, a sixty-two-year-old patient of Malissa, recalls how phone calls from her difficult daughter would routinely lead her to the pantry or refrigerator. These angst-filled moments would often result in her eating a whole loaf of bread or box of cookies. So when she sought help from Malissa and her team, one of the first steps they took together was to examine the routines that Kelly would engage in when she experienced emotional stress—behaviors she was not even entirely aware of at the time. Once the emotional triggers behind her habits were revealed, Kelly finally recognized that the behaviors were linked.

It sounds simple. But in the moments that we are stressed, scared, or anxious, it can be difficult to recognize the connection. Most important, once this connection between emotion and behavior became clear to Kelly,

Malissa's Story:

GETTING OUT OF THE COMFORT FOOD "COMFORT ZONE"

Our relationship with food develops early in life. While we may learn as small children that the extra peanut butter and jelly sandwich in the lunch box helps ease the anxiety associated with the first day of school, our bodies' response to this learned and consistently reinforced behavior changes with age. While I could pull off the extra sandwich without a second thought in seventh grade, or the box of Ritz crackers sitting on my desk while I studied for my boards in medical school, these choices would certainly lead to an expanding waistline later on in life. I really noticed the effect this behavior had on my weight during internship. Suddenly I was working long hours, I was not getting much sleep or exercise, and I was really looking forward to my breaks at breakfast, lunch, dinner, and snack time. I started internship at 24 years of age weighing 132 pounds. By the middle of my intern year, I had hit the 144 mark.

I thought about my approach and decided it was time to make a change. I bought a pair of running shoes and hit the pavement. I would go for runs after work and on weekends and found that not only did running help me manage my stress, but it also helped me manage my weight. Before I knew it, I was back on track.

she developed strategies to defuse her negative routine. Sometimes this meant dispatching her daughter to voice mail if she knew that picking up her call would lead to stress, or taking a walk around the block instead of to the fridge in response to a heated argument. Ultimately, for Kelly, these and other small changes had a large impact: a weight loss of thirty pounds over the next year.

Inner-Self Factor #3: Food Addiction

The third inner factor is unique in that it relates closely to both physiology and psychology. Although scientists are still debating whether it should be called an addiction, much recent evidence documents that specific foods can generate responses in the brain similar to those seen with addictive drugs.[11] Like other addictions, food addiction—the act of using food as a drug—can be triggered by certain emotional events. And some researchers are beginning to shed light on genes that make many of us more susceptible to food addiction.

In addition to the possibility we can become addicted to food, eating sweet, starchy, fatty, or salty foods can trigger the cascade of chemical reactions in the brain that lead to a "reward" signal. At the center of this reward system is a chemical in the brain called dopamine. You may have heard of dopamine. Simply put, it is the chemical messenger in the brain that is a crucial part of the chemical reactions that lead to reward and pleasure. Drugs like cocaine become addictive because they cause the brain to be flooded with dopamine. And this same chemical system can be activated for some people by consuming certain foods. As evidence of how similar these reactions in the brain can be, Harvard researcher Dr. David Ludwig showed in a recent article in the *American Journal of Clinical Nutrition* that foods with a high glycemic index—those that cause the blood sugar to spike—actually increase bloodflow to the same areas of the brain activated by addictive drugs.[12]

For some people, this reward signal leads to a chronic disorder. They fall into a pattern of behavior in which they impulsively seek out the foods that give them this "high." With food addiction, satisfying this impulse transcends emotional eating—it becomes a persistent and recurrent urge.

Researchers at the Yale Rudd Center for Food Policy and Obesity have developed a tool to assess the presence of food addiction, known as the Yale Food Addiction Scale.[13] The tool is a series of questions, of which a few are below. Take a quick look—do any of these sound familiar?

Your Emotional Eating Emergency Kit

At one point or another, everyone has engaged in some form of emotional eating. It's a natural reaction to stress. Walter, who has a great deal of experience writing book chapters under the gun, admits that at times he, too, oversnacked when he was stressed over a looming deadline.

Avoiding the urge to eat when stressed out 100 percent of the time would truly be a feat of willpower. The trick, then, is to be prepared when the temptation strikes. Walter's solution? A convenient and accessible emotional eating emergency kit that contains healthier options than the foods for which you normally would have reached. The following are just a few options you can include in case the urge to munch on something strikes:

◊ Apples
◊ Cut and sliced raw vegetables
◊ Air-popped popcorn
◊ Hard-boiled eggs
◊ Whole wheat crackers
◊ Whole grain, high-fiber cereal
◊ Dark chocolate (in moderation)

For Walter, the proof came during his work on various editions of his textbook on nutritional epidemiology. Writing the first edition—and snacking on cookies while he did—led to five extra pounds that took a while to lose. The second edition, which was even longer but was written with lots of carrots and apples nearby, led to no weight gain and many nutritional benefits.

IN THE PAST 12 MONTHS:

◊ When I start eating certain foods, I end up eating much more than I had planned.

◊ There have been times when I consumed certain foods so often or in such large quantities that I spent time dealing with negative feelings from overeating instead of working, spending time with my family or friends, or engaging in other important activities or recreational activities I enjoy.

◊ Over time, I have found that I need to eat more and more to get the feeling I want, such as reduced negative emotions or increased pleasure.

◊ I have had withdrawal symptoms when I cut down or stopped eating certain foods (aside from caffeinated beverages). For example: developing physical symptoms, feeling agitated, or feeling anxious.

◊ I experience significant problems in my ability to function effectively (daily routine, job/school, social activities, family activities, health difficulties) because of food and eating.

If these sound familiar to you, it is possible that you have some level of food addiction. The first thing you should do is realize that you are not alone. In 2012, a team of researchers led by Alan J. Flint, MD, DrPH, examined the answers to the questionnaire provided by middle-age and older women in two large ongoing studies—the Nurses' Health Study and the Nurses' Health Study II—for a total of more than 134,000 women. Dr. Flint and colleagues found that 5.8 percent of the women surveyed provided answers that identified them as having a food addiction.[14] In the younger of the two groups of women studied—those age forty-five to sixty-four—this percentage was 8.4 percent.

Not surprisingly, these researchers determined that meeting the criteria for a food addiction was directly related to being heavier, even within a BMI range considered normal. Specifically, women with BMIs of 35 or greater were 15 to 18 times more likely to report symptoms of food addiction compared to women with a BMI between 18.5 and 22.9.

Ongoing research is exploring the extent to which genetic factors contribute to food addiction, and it is likely that genes do play some role.[15] But just like other common addictions such as those related to caffeine and tobacco, having such an addiction does not mean your fate is sealed. What it does mean, in the context of our Thinfluence approach, is that you may be dealing with a strong inner factor that will affect your relationship with all of the other circles of your life and will, in turn, affect your weight. Bringing addiction under control may not be easy at first, but fortunately counselors who are well trained in dealing with all forms of addiction can help. The important thing to remember is that food addictions, like the other inner factors we have discussed, are within the innermost area of our Circles of Influence graph (page 10) for a reason. Ultimately—and sometimes with a certain measure of outside help—we can control these things directly. And the more control we have over our inner factors, the more success we have in dealing with the other areas of our lives and their effects on our weight.

Are Inner-Self Factors All about You?

As we have just discussed, inner factors can have a powerful effect on your ability to achieve or maintain the weight you want for yourself. But these factors are not all about you. No person is an island, and we can likewise see that even the factors we view as within our innermost circle of influence do not act in isolation.

Consider food addiction. We know about the circuits in the brain that, when activated, reinforce the feelings of reward and comfort that come with certain foods. But if we take a step back, we can see the advertising and marketing environment that exploits our vulnerabilities and encourages the development of these problems.

The psychological factors that form the basis for emotional eating often seem remarkably individualized—so much so that they can be isolating for the people who experience them. However, a complex web of social and familial interactions and relationships often play an important contributing role in the strong emotions involved.

And we know we can't change the genes that stack the deck against our efforts to attain a healthier weight. But the features of the day-to-day environments where we live go a long way in determining the foods we consume and the level of physical activity we get—which together have a more dramatic impact on our weight than does the genetic hand we are dealt.

In short, while it is important to understand "inner-self" factors regarding weight, we must not stop there. And to get started, it is key to understand the ways that our environment and the multitude of external factors we encounter in our daily lives affect our sense of personal responsibility in weight control.

Walter, along with his colleague Kelly Brownell, PhD, analyzed this very issue in 2010—specifically, how personal responsibility is framed in the context of social, legal, and political approaches to obesity. All too often, they noted in their report published in the journal *Health Affairs*,[16] the social, legal, and political approaches to overweight and obesity tend to neglect the importance of environmental conditions with regard to the problem. As a result, obesity is overwhelmingly viewed as an individual failure to be responsible, an attitude that creates an overriding sense of stigma for those who are struggling with their weight.

Thinfluence Action Plan: Tackling Your Inner-Self Factors

Hopefully this chapter has given you a better understanding of the various factors that may be contributing to your weight so you can develop a framework for dealing with them. These factors may be related to your diet and activity, but they may also have social, psychological, and emotional components. And though these factors are personal, you will likely see that they, too, can depend strongly upon external influences.

But it is important to realize that your inner factors, if properly tuned, can help you send your positive influence outward, too, into other areas of your life. Many broader changes, after all, begin with one individual. Could you be the person who brings more positive weight-related behaviors to the people and environments in your life? It could happen. And taking control of your inner factors is the first step.

As you have been reading, you may have found yourself thinking about the inner factors that have the biggest impact on your weight. As you proceed through the Thinfluence Action Plan exercise below, you will be able to put some of this new knowledge into practice.

ANALYZE

1. To what extent have relatives experienced the same struggles with weight that you have?

    A. Weight issues definitely run in my family. Both of my parents, as well as other members of my immediate family, seem to be at risk of unhealthy weight.

    B. My family does seem to have a bit of a history of weight problems, but some members of my family—siblings, a parent, or children—have never seemed to have a serious problem with weight.

    C. Most, if not all, of my immediate family members appear to be genetically blessed when it comes to their weight.

2. What is your emotional state currently—in other words, how do you feel from day to day?

    A. Honestly speaking, I am a naturally stressed/anxious/depressed person. When things get touchy, these emotional factors weigh down on me even more heavily.

    B. It varies, but I do feel that there are times when stress, anxiety, or simply "having the blues" takes a toll on how I feel. I do feel that I am at least somewhat susceptible to these emotions when the going gets tough.

C. Even though I am not free from worry, I feel that emotionally
speaking I can deal with problems that arise in my life very
effectively, without getting too stressed out, anxious, or depressed.

3. To what extent do you feel your emotions are tied to the choices
relating to the healthfulness of your lifestyle?

A. There is a very close connection. When I am emotionally distressed,
it is difficult to muster up the motivation to eat well, exercise, or
engage in other healthy behaviors.

B. My state of mind is connected to my behaviors at least some of the
time. But occasional emotional challenges are usually not enough
to completely derail the healthy aspects of my routine.

C. I don't let my emotions undermine the healthy choices I make.

ACT

Take a look at your responses to the questions. How did you score?

◊ Mostly As: It is likely that your inner factors are playing a very
important role in your weight. While this may seem discouraging at
first, it is actually very powerful information. It means that your
starting point should be in recognizing how these inner factors
relate to your weight and taking steps to deal with them. For some
inner factors, like a genetic risk for obesity, the most important
thing you can do is realize that changes to your habits and lifestyle
can mitigate the impact of these genes. If emotional issues seem to
be more important for you, the first step lies in dealing with the
root causes of these issues and making sure you are aware of how
your emotions may be impacting your eating and exercise habits.

◊ Mostly Bs: For most everyone, inner factors play some role in
weight. The important thing is to know which of these factors have

the most influence on the actions you take in other areas of your life that impact your weight.

◊ Mostly Cs: While it appears that inner factors may have less of an impact on your weight than do other factors outside of your direct control, it is important to be aware of how your emotions and other inner factors might be interacting with other areas of your life. As you read further, you may be surprised to find that they matter more than you initially believed.

INFLUENCE

What positive outcomes can result from the choices you can share with those around you to influence their behaviors? Here are a few examples:

◊ Improved emotional health

◊ Weight loss and better fitness

◊ Less stress and anxiety, both with regard to family interactions and your weight and self-image

◊ Leading by example and demonstrating to your friends and family that the challenges you may be facing in your life—both in and out of your control—don't have to torpedo your efforts at living a healthier life

◊ Taking stock of areas that need work and dealing with them directly sends a strong message to those around you that you have made a commitment to a healthier life and you are working from the inside out.

You may find that you can use these positive outcomes to motivate those closest to you to support you in the changes you are making—and maybe even influence them to make changes of their own.

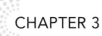

CHAPTER 3

Family Matters: How Your Closest Relationships Affect Your Weight

"The dose makes the poison."

It is a phrase coined by the Renaissance physician Paracelsus hundreds of years ago. And while you might not hear it every day, it's popular among toxicologists, whose job it is to study the effects of exposure to unhealthy substances in our physical environment. But it also rings true for our exposure to messages, routines, and other influences within our *social* environment. And this "exposure" is arguably the greatest when the source lives with us in our homes.

For many of us, the biggest dose of this influence comes from our family. These closest relationships hold the greatest sway over our ability to practice healthy diet and exercise habits.

And if this influence is "toxic"—if it involves unhealthy social pressures or behaviors—it can greatly affect your chances of achieving the weight you want. Take Miriam, a fifty-three-year-old patient of Malissa at the HAPPY Heart clinic, who'd had an unhealthy relationship with food since she was a teenager. Although she had once been petite and at a healthy weight, she had never been "thin" enough for her father when she was younger. In addition, Miriam's mother had always been very particular about food, insisting that certain things be eaten in certain combinations.

"My father and his family were obsessed with weight," she recalls. "If you weren't thin, you weren't going to amount to anything. I constantly heard that I'd never meet a man or get a good job. I never felt that I was good enough."

The constant negative messages and criticism took their toll. They eroded Miriam's self-esteem—and that, combined with her mother's rigid beliefs, led her to become fixated on food. "I remember going to the refrigerator and looking inside and thinking, 'I can't wait until I grow up and have my own fridge, and I can eat anything I want.' And when I grew up and moved out, that's exactly what I did. Whenever I was stressed or unhappy, food was my escape. It made me feel good."

Not surprisingly, this "escape" led Miriam to gain weight. She married a man who in retrospect she realized was as focused on her weight as her father had been—yet another close family relationship that contributed to her unhealthy relationship with food. By the time she came to see Malissa at the clinic, she weighed 198 pounds. She knew she needed to make a change, but she also knew that simply going on a "diet" was not going to be enough to address the underlying causes of her unhealthy weight.

Miriam's story illustrates how family relationships can be a catalyst for a weight problem. She may have had control over her diet, her activity levels, and other inner factors, but until she addressed the effects of her family relationships, her battle against an unhealthy weight would continue to be uphill.

But just as the dose can make the poison, in Miriam's case it also made the cure.

The "Family Effect" and What It Means for Your Weight

You probably realized long ago that certain personality attributes and behavior patterns are essentially unspoken cues you have inherited from those closest to you. When people live or otherwise spend a lot of time together, their common environment creates a huge opportunity for shared behaviors and mentalities regarding a number of things, not the least of which are food, weight, and lifestyle.

The first step, then, is to learn how to recognize the different attitudes that prevail in families and understand how they impact your weight. One way to do this is to decode the "archetypes" within your family—the common patterns of behavior that can help explain why certain family members act the way they do when it comes to food, exercise, and healthy lifestyle changes. Once you have a better understanding of these patterns, you might even begin to see how your own influence within your family fits in and how you can change this for the better.

Decoding Your Family "Archetypes"

Certain personality types or roles are very influential on a family's weight for a number of reasons. Among the most important of these is the fact that attitudes can be infectious, especially if the person expressing them happens to be a leader or authority figure within the family. Once these attitudes spread within the family and are accepted as the "norm" in the home, they can shape the behaviors of everyone going forward.

Because of this, changing the established daily patterns of those you love can be a challenge, and it is crucial to determine what your role is in your family's choices with regard to behaviors and routines that can pack on the pounds and make weight loss difficult. Of course, many of us already have roles that we play within our families: mother or father, sister or brother. You may play the role of a leader within your family, or you may follow the rest and offer support.

One important point is to be made regarding these archetypes: They are meant only for characterization, not as a guide for where to point the finger of blame. Finding out which of these models helps explain your behavior and identifying the role that others in your family may be playing helps start the conversation that will hopefully lead to where the problem lies within your family.

•••THE TRADITIONALIST•••
COMMON QUOTE: "I like my meat and potatoes, and I'm not willing to sacrifice them."

The traditionalist views food as a constant, a ritual. For this person, there is comfort in routine—whether that routine is healthy or not. If this person has a high degree of influence within the family, and if their preferences are unhealthy, their mentality toward food is an anchor that can weigh the rest of the family down, keeping them away from improvements in diet and health.

IF YOUR FAMILY HAS ONE:
Changing the established daily patterns of those you love can be no small task, but it is possible. It might help to start by trying to recognize and acknowledge the food-related family traditions in your household and determine why this family member places so much importance on them. Keep in mind that if this person is so committed to preserving the family routines he or she sees as important, it is also likely that they have a strong commitment to the family in other ways as well. Use this to your advantage; let this person know how his or her choices are affecting the family— and how a change in their mentality toward healthy food can have a big payoff in terms of improved health, weight, and quality of life for the ones they love the most.

IF *YOU* ARE THE TRADITIONALIST:
If you are calling the shots at the dinner table, you probably wield a great deal of influence at home. It is especially important for you to understand the impact of your preferences, not only on you but on your loved ones as well. The next is to realize that you have the power to change the patterns

you have set for your family. Is it possible to keep the tradition but modify it? Perhaps spaghetti Fridays could benefit from less meat and more diced vegetables in the sauce. Maybe it's also time to start some new traditions—ones that emphasize fresh foods, whole grains, and vegetables and discourage processed foods or those chock-full of saturated fat or empty calories.

···THE GIFTEDLY THIN···

COMMON QUOTE: "You can do your thing; I'm not the one with the problem."

Every family has one—the sibling, parent, or spouse who seems to be able to eat anything he or she wants, skip the gym, and still never put on an ounce. In some cases, this person's appearance may be an inspiration to other family members. He or she may even be the only one who adheres to a healthy lifestyle. Alternatively, this person's ability to keep the weight off can be discouraging to others around them, particularly if their enviable weight is not obviously the result of diet or lifestyle factors. In the worst cases, these individuals may behave as though they do not need to control what they eat or what they do.

IF YOUR FAMILY HAS ONE:

As tempting as it may be, try not to compare yourself to this individual. Everyone faces their own challenges with their weight; for some it is just more obvious than it is for others. The other key is not to be discouraged. Talk to this family member; see if they will agree to support you and be your "cheerleader" as you try to attain a better weight for yourself. The way to start this conversation is to tell this relative what your goals are—that you would like to achieve a healthier weight—and that you would like them to hold you accountable to a better diet and more activity. Even if the giftedly thin person in your family does not exhibit any overt behaviors that have led to a better weight, do what you can to emulate them, matching their portion size at the dinner table or accompanying them when they are enjoying some kind of physical activity. Most important, do what you can to get them on board with your cause. Having this person as part of the effort—whether it is for you individually or for the family as a whole—can be a huge asset when making a healthy change in your lifestyle.

IF *YOU* ARE THE GIFTEDLY THIN:

Chances are, you are reading this book on behalf of your family rather than for yourself. You may have already been trying to get your spouse or children to eat healthier, but your efforts aren't paying off in the way you hoped they would. It can be difficult for people who struggle with their weight to hear advice from someone who maintains a healthy weight without much obvious effort. No matter how delicately you think you are phrasing your comments, they can be interpreted as criticism rather than concern. Another stumbling block may be that you and the other slender family members eat one way but expect the people who need to lose weight to eat another way. One solution to both problems is for everyone in the family to eat the same meals and to center those meals on lean protein, whole grains, low-fat dairy, vegetables, and fruit. Explain the changes in the family's eating habits in terms of overall health rather than weight, and stress that everyone can benefit from a healthy diet. If a family member needs more energy—if one child is very active, for instance—that person can have bigger portions. Minimize the chips, crackers, ice cream, and soda in the house. It's not realistic to expect only the slender people to eat them, and in any case too much of these foods is not healthy for anyone of any size.

• • •THE NURTURER• • •
COMMON QUOTE: "You look like you need a second helping. And save room for pie!"

The nurturer shows love with food, and a great deal of it. While this person is typically viewed as a mom whose apple pie or pot roast is the stuff of family legend, they can really be anyone—the father who loves to cook gourmet, the uncle who lights up the grill whenever the weather is warm, the daughter who loves to watch people eat her "famous" cupcakes—as long as they have the power to influence their family to eat and snack more.

IF YOUR FAMILY HAS ONE:

Tread carefully. For this member of your family, food is the way they show their love. Of course, showing love with food is far from uncommon. In a 2013 nationally representative poll by NPR, the Robert Wood Johnson Foundation, and the Harvard School of Public Health, researchers found that more than a quarter of parents agreed that enjoying tasty foods high in fat and sugar was "an important way [their family] shows affection."[1] The nurturer views himself or herself as the source of this love—it is, literally and figuratively, what they bring to the table. So to many nurturers, saying no or pushing away from the table can be interpreted as pushing away their love. If someone in your family fits the description of a nurturer, you have a choice, other than eating everything they push your way. It is more important to remember that there are ways for you to show appreciation for the food other than eating all of it. Tell them it is delicious, but be honest and firm when you say that you could not eat another bite. Remind them even away from the dinner table how much you love their cooking. The nurturer is after the feeling that they have done something for you, that they have given you and the rest of your family an experience everyone has enjoyed, so express that appreciation.

IF *YOU* ARE THE NURTURER:

The fact that you show your love with food probably means, in turn, that your family loves your food. This is not always a bad thing. But realize that your position as the family's favorite cook comes with a great deal of responsibility. If you make your family feel as if they are rejecting you when they refuse second or third helpings, you are setting them up for behaviors they could later regret. If there are children in your family, you have the power to shape their tastes and appetite not only at home, but also their food preferences and habits outside of the home. Challenge yourself to create dishes that are not only tasty, but also nutritious and healthful. And learn to listen to those three *other* little words from your loved ones: "I'm full, thanks!"

···THE PICKY EATER···
COMMON QUOTE: "I don't like that. Where's the pizza?"

While one might not think that a picky child—or a picky adult for that matter—would have so much influence over an entire family's eating patterns, it only takes having one in the household to understand his or her true impact. On one hand, there is the threat of every meal turning into a minefield of negotiation. On the other, there is a real possibility that the whole family will be eating pepperoni pizza and macaroni and cheese for three days straight. Either way, it is highly likely that one or more parties will leave the table feeling unsatisfied with the situation, unless you count the pizza guy. Worst, picky kids often grow up to be picky adults, and they influence what their spouses and their children eat and are exposed to.

IF YOUR FAMILY HAS ONE:
There are a number of ways to defuse the situation before the food even hits the table, especially where kids are concerned. Why not make choosing recipes a family activity? Getting picky kids involved with food choices and preparation allows them to see what they are eating before they eat it—and it may even help them generate a sense of pride in helping to create the family meal. Often the more a child understands about what he or she is eating, the more likely they will eat and enjoy it. You can even have fun with this by integrating it into other aspects of the child's life. One way to do this, for example, is to find out what culture your child is studying in geography class and try to serve healthy traditional dishes from that area. Think about the healthy foods that people eat in those countries and try to replicate them. All of this is to say that as you strive to help the picky kid eat a healthier, more diverse diet, you may find the challenge to be fun as well.

IF *YOU* ARE THE PICKY EATER:

As we alluded to earlier, not all picky eaters are children. While adults are far less likely to throw a tantrum at the dinner table if they see a food they do not like, they also wield much more power in determining the daily menu. If the pickiness you developed as a child has persisted, it is quite possible that your food likes and dislikes will dictate what everyone eats. So the first thing you must realize is that your hang-ups about food affect the health and weight of others in your family. If you find that your pickiness is more of a preference—in other words, if you are only *slightly* finicky—try setting goals for yourself to try two or three new foods every week. Start with foods that are somewhat similar to the ones you already enjoy, making sure to lean toward healthier options whenever possible. But if you find that your food fixations are more serious, you may try seeking help from a therapist to help you overcome this issue. Remember, you exert an influence on your family whether you know it or not. Why not make sure it is positive?

···THE SHRUGGER···
COMMON QUOTE: "Look, we're just a heavy family.
It's in our genes. Why fight it?"

The shrugger is resistant to any kind of change in the routine, regardless of the potential health benefits. In many cases, this person is the "anti-influence"—not actively motivating his or her family members to adopt new unhealthy behaviors, but at the same time bringing a defeatist attitude to efforts to make healthy changes. And while the shrugger may view themselves as neutral within the family's health-related decisions, they may be exerting more of an influence than they think in their unwillingness to make changes to the status quo.

IF YOUR FAMILY HAS ONE:

The shrugger may not seem interested in getting on board with the healthy changes you are suggesting for your family—at least not at first. This is a

situation where actions may speak louder than words. The key to changing his or her attitude is to show him or her the changes in yourself and other members of your family. Once you show this person that healthy changes are possible, that being overweight isn't a genetic destiny to which the whole family is doomed, it's likely that he or she will be enthusiastic in joining the cause.

IF *YOU* ARE THE SHRUGGER:

It's a fact: Change is hard! And it's possible you feel that when your family tries to make a healthy change, it is a change that you have tried to make before, unsuccessfully. So it is understandable that you may be feeling less than enthused when a family member tries to get everyone else on board for some lifestyle tweaks that could mean you will be eating differently, exercising more, or altering some other aspect of day-to-day life. But it is important to realize that your reluctance to support your loved ones may be throwing a bucket of cold water on their enthusiasm for ideas that could end up helping everyone attain a less obesogenic, healthier lifestyle. At some point it may be time to face the fact that some changes really can happen—and you can be a part of them.

···THE AUDIENCE MEMBER···
COMMON QUOTE: "You go ahead and eat your salad and go on your run—I'm proud of you! Meanwhile I'm going to have my steak and watch TV, if you don't mind."

The person who sits on the couch while you are out running or who orders a burger and fries while you have a salad really believes that he or she is supporting your healthy efforts. But they are often the ones who continue to stock the pantry with boxes of tempting snack cakes. Chances are, they do not even realize they are dampening the resolve of their spouse or sibling who is striving to lose a few pounds—even when

the evidence is right in front of them in the form of a thick slice of chocolate cake.

IF YOUR FAMILY HAS ONE:
When dealing with an audience member, it is important to emphasize the spirit of the support they have expressed while bringing to their attention the ways they may be sabotaging the efforts of those around them. It probably will not help to get angry with them or express your disappointment; remember that in their minds, they could be the very model of a supportive family member! But gently pointing out what they are doing when they are doing it could help them recognize the effect they are having—and it may even get them to adopt some of the healthier lifestyle changes of those around them.

IF *YOU* ARE THE AUDIENCE MEMBER:
You may sincerely hope that the changes one or more of the people in your family are making help them attain the weight they want. But now your actions must reflect this hope—at the very least when you are around them. Support them in actions, not just in words. They will appreciate it, and you may even find that you are healthier for it yourself.

Thinfluence Action Plan: Engaging with Your Family

A series of small changes can make a big difference. On the food front, maybe this means sneaking in a bit of whole grains to substitute for white rice or slowly increasing the amount of vegetables in your most popular sauce recipes. For physical activity, perhaps it means that one night a week you unplug the television and go for a walk instead. You may not be able to change everything at once—and that's okay!

ANALYZE

1. How do you and your family eat?

   A. The kitchen or dining room table is rarely used; most of our meals take place in front of the TV. Family meals together are pretty rare—usually, it's every man for himself. As far as food choices go, healthfulness and nutrition usually take a backseat to convenience.

   B. We do our best to have at least several meals per week together, though busy schedules sometimes make this difficult. When we do eat together, we try to make it a "real" dinner experience, with nutritious fare and few extraneous distractions.

   C. Family meals are the norm in our house, and we strive to make conversation and healthy foods the centerpiece of our time together.

2. What part does physical activity play in your time with your family?

   A. We get little, if any, regular physical activity. Any effort to get more exercise is usually an individual undertaking and is usually short-lived.

   B. There have been times in the past when our family has gone on a "health kick." While these have rarely led to lasting lifestyle changes, a few people in my family have made improvements in their weight through these efforts.

   C. Physical activity is a priority in our family. Exercising together involves everyone, and we have shared in the benefits as well!

3. When it comes to healthy lifestyle changes, to what extent would you say your family is "on board"?

A. It's a real challenge to get everyone on the same page. I feel that if I were to bring up the idea of a healthy new regimen, regardless of whether it involved food or activity, I would have a very hard time getting everyone on board.

B. I feel that my family members are generally supportive of healthy lifestyle changes, but they are not very likely to join in or stick with changes over the long term. There are no "saboteurs" in the ranks, but there aren't any strong advocates either.

C. My family is primed and ready to go. Not only would they be supportive of healthy lifestyle changes, but they would be enthused to create the supportive family environment that would help a new regimen last.

4. How confident are you in your own ability to motivate your family to take steps toward a more weight-friendly lifestyle?

A. I would find it difficult to motivate my family to change their routine. I may fall into one of the family "archetype" categories that have been a roadblock to healthy changes for myself and my family in the past.

B. I may be able to help my family embark on some of the first steps toward a lifestyle that leads to a better weight. I may not be the leader of the family, but I feel like I could leverage my influence to make some positive changes happen.

C. I am absolutely confident that my efforts will make a difference in my family's weight and health. I feel that I would not only be able to get the momentum going, but also set an example for those closest to me.

ACT

Review your answers to these questions. How do your responses pan out?

◊ Mostly As: Don't despair. This is the starting point at which many people find themselves with their families. Perhaps the best first step you can take is to find one or two members of your family who you feel would stand behind you in the efforts to instill a new set of

Family Traditions: Helping or Hindering a Healthy Weight?

Nearly every family has an eating "tradition." Whether or not that actual term is used, it is clear that certain time-honored practices go along with food. These are perhaps most obvious during occasions like holidays—the Thanksgiving turkey, the Easter ham. But truthfully, your family food traditions also include what happens from day to day.

Some of these traditions are excessive. The fact is that the culinary tradition of the United States is an animal-based diet, incorporating such elements as lard and butter. These offerings were often the only choices available to our ancestors and their cold-weather agricultural system. They did not eat these patently unhealthy foods out of ignorance of healthy food—it was simply out of necessity. Unfortunately, many of these traditions have been "baked into" the food traditions that families have today—ones that can lead to unhealthy weight gain unless you happen to be plowing a field or hauling buckets of milk every morning.

On the other hand, other family traditions can benefit your health and weight. Before modern methods of refrigeration and food processing were available, people in many cultures practiced the art of eating seasonally, building their cuisines around the foods that weight-friendly norms. This group approach could create a better environment for changes to stick, and these family advocates will also help you stay on track even in challenging times.

◊ Mostly Bs: It sounds like you have some good things going for you in terms of your own influence and your family dynamics. Using the advice we have provided in this chapter, you might start making some small changes that are likely to stick. Don't try to make

happened to be available during a particular time of the year. Numerous foods have become traditional seasonal ones that people don't seem to eat anymore—cabbage, root vegetables, parsnips. All of these nutritious foods can be added to your family's seasonal menu, perhaps allowing you to avoid some of the more processed and less healthy options out there.

Behavioral traditions related to culture can also have a huge impact on eating patterns. In cultures for whom hardship has been a hallmark in the past, there may be a strong admonition to "clean your plate" or "eat the potatoes"— after all, you never know when food is not going to be there. This "survival mode" thinking is good advice for a famine, but not so applicable when you live around as many calories as Americans do

today. Unfortunately, many people have incorporated this principle as a green light for eating anything they want.

If your family's ethnic heritage is reflected in the food you prepare in your home, bear in mind that every culture has its healthy and unhealthy options. The Mediterranean diet, for example—whose name has been appropriated by all means of high-carb, high-fat foods in popular restaurants—is actually one of the healthiest cuisines in the world in its purest form. The trick is to take what works in a given ethnic tradition and apply it, while leaving out what does not.

Food means something special, and traditions have a reason behind them. It's up to you and your family to pick the traditions that provide the healthiest approach.

too many changes at once; focus on generating some momentum first. Once others in your family start to see better numbers on the scale themselves, they will be more likely to build on the foundation you have established.

◊ Mostly Cs: You are in an enviable situation in the family department. The question that you should be asking yourself at this point is, why haven't I already started these changes? The answer may lead you to the surprising conclusion that you are the one in your family who may be missing out on the healthy opportunities that already exist within your closest social circle. Make sure you take advantage of your excellent family support system, and you are very likely to succeed in your goals.

Regardless of your responses, you can start a number of small steps right away to give you and your family a push in the right direction. Here are just a few ideas:

◊ Educate your loved ones about the potential land mines of bad food and beverage choices out there; if you don't, they may not learn this anywhere else. It's not like we walk into a fast-food chain and there is a warning sign over the door. By providing just a little bit of information in a straightforward, nonthreatening manner, you may, over the course of time, have an impact on your family's food choices outside of the home. Resolve to improve your own knowledge base on healthy eating issues by the end of the week, either by referring to books on the topic or visiting reputable Web sites. By the end of the month, you should have enough information to share with your family.

◊ Cook at home, and make it a colorful and fun family activity. Offer fresh vegetables as an appetizer, engage the family in choosing toppings for their whole wheat pasta, let each member of the family select the menu for one meal during the week, and, even better, ask them to help with the preparation. Instead of fast food, substitute healthier meals made in a slow cooker that take just about the same amount of time and just a little extra effort. Turn it into a game—have a competition in which family members on different days strive to create the most healthful, delicious meal they can for the rest of the family. Make it a point to prepare at least one meal you normally would not by the end of the week. It may be easier than you think. Your goal for the end of the month should be to establish a schedule by which you and your family are eating at least three more healthy, home-prepared meals a week than you would otherwise.

◊ Simply don't purchase food you know you and your family should not eat. Chances are, if you buy it you will eat it. Stock up on healthier snack options and minimize the high-sugar and highly refined carbohydrate products that come in packages. Your goal for the end of the week should be to complete a grocery shopping trip without reaching for any of these options. In addition, take inventory of the unhealthy food options in your home. Once you have this inventory, resolve to cut this list down by at least half by the end of the month. It may be easier than you think!

◊ Put those extra-large plates away in storage and save them for a special occasion. Purchase small to medium-size dinner plates for daily use. Studies have shown that larger plates actually lead us to eat more in a single sitting.[2,3]

◊ Encourage your family to engage in lively discussion during dinner. By actually taking the time for conversation, you will likely slow down your eating, end up feeling fuller without eating as much, and save yourself a few hundred calories by passing on that second helping.

◊ Teach your kids (or possibly your spouse) to read a label and understand fat, whether it is saturated or trans fat; recommended daily allowances of various nutrients; calories; and serving sizes. Start modestly; aim to explain to them the concept of calories, fat, and sodium by the end of the week. Your goal is to instill within your family a working knowledge of how to separate healthy options from less healthy ones, which should be doable within a month.

◊ Engage the help of a professional. Nutritionists are magicians! They can take dishes that are traditional in your family, culture, or

How Cost Matters in a Family's Diet

For the majority of families, a factor at play when it comes to healthy decisions at the dinner table is cost.

The reason it makes sense to think about this is because there is a very real connection between the cost of food and the likelihood that it will make you and your family fat. In 2005, a study in the *American Journal of Clinical Nutrition* showed just that; specifically, researchers compared what they called the "energy density" of foods to their cost per calorie.[4] They found that the foods with the lowest cost per calorie also contain overly refined grains as well as added sugar.

Healthier, more nutritious foods, such as fish, fruits, and vegetables, are usually pricier.

In short, the healthier food is, the more it usually costs.

Unfortunately, much of this situation is largely out of your control; after all, you don't set the price at the grocery store, nor are you in charge of the political and economic environment that sets the stage for high-calorie, processed foods to be more affordable than healthier options. In later chapters we will look at what you can do with regard to these factors—but you will be happy to know that you can operate in other ways region and help you transform them into healthier versions. If you can't afford a nutritionist or a health coach.

◊ Start encouraging your family to make exercise a priority. Find a few subtle ways to incorporate just a little more exercise into the family routine, and stick with them.

within your own household's budget to overcome this.

Instead of red meat, try nuts as a protein source: Fish can be expensive. Swapping in nuts and seeds can often give you almost as much protein per ounce, often at half the cost or less. If you are curious about how you can incorporate them into a meal, many recipes are available from which to choose.

Choose basic ingredients over pre-prepared foods: In general, the more prepared a food is when we buy it, the more it costs. Instead of going for the pre-prepared version of a food, think about basic ingredients—whole grains, certain vegetables, and other ingredients. You will probably find that many of these healthy ingredients cost very little compared to their more prepared

counterparts. Sure, it may take a bit more time and effort to prepare meals using these ingredients. But you will also find that this approach gives you more control; it lets you know exactly what's going into your dinner, which is yet another way to cut the calories while boosting nutrients.

Consider growing your own vegetables: Are costs at the grocery store pricing you out of fresh, healthy vegetables? You might try starting your own home or community garden. If you have the space (and it may take less space than you think), as well as the inclination, you may end up with a steady supply of seasonal, fresh vegetables year-round—just one way that your green thumb may save you a bit of green as well.

By this time, you have probably considered at least a few steps you can take or strategies you can employ to encourage the lifestyle changes in your family that will help lead all of you to a better weight. In the example we have created, even setting a few of these adjustments into motion can have big benefits. Here are some potential outcomes that you can use to help motivate yourself, as well as those in your family, to take those healthy steps and stick to them:

◊ Improved diet choices, leading to a better weight for you and your family

◊ Better financial health as a result of preparing more food at home and breaking out of the fast-food, junk food, and prepared food routine

◊ Greater family harmony and togetherness through new, healthier routines and activities

◊ Cultivation of a lifelong understanding of healthy eating, fostering early lifestyle changes in your children that can have big dividends

Making Healthy Weight a Family Affair

The key to using relationships to solve these problems is engagement. If you don't engage with your family, you are not going to realize how the decisions made on the individual and group levels influence your chances of a better weight and a healthier lifestyle. Being a bystander in this area of your life—choosing not to speak up if you see a problem—enables your family to make bad decisions.

Of course, we know that it is not always easy to talk to your family about this. The trick is to advise them without haranguing them. A number of strategies may soften the blow of the suggestion that a change is necessary. It may help some members of your family if they get that information from another source, such as an informative book. Direct conflict is rarely the answer, so it is wise to approach the matter with care and understanding.

For Miriam, whom we discussed at the opening of this chapter, being a bystander when she had her own family to raise was not an option. Individually she has made great strides. She divorced her husband eight years ago—a step she says helped her overcome many of the psychological issues she faced with regard to her weight since her childhood. Over the past year and a half, she has lost forty-five pounds, and today she describes herself as a size 8, in good shape at 150 pounds.

She still finds strength in her older family relationships as well. Her brother, who Miriam says has never struggled with weight, nonetheless has been one of her strongest sources of support in her own weight battles.

"Even at my heaviest, he never put me down for it," she says. "He's just amazing . . . he's very supportive."

But the change that is most important to Miriam is not the weight she has lost. It is the positive attitudes about weight and health that she never had in her younger life, but which she has managed to instill in her children. Her two children are now young adults. Both, she says, are very fit; her daughter is a part-time policewoman, while her son works at a gym.

"They got the gym rat gene I didn't," she says with a smile. "And I remember saying, 'I'm never going to put them down for food, never going to try to control their food.'"

What would Miriam do if she could go back and talk to the teenage girl she was forty years ago, when she was navigating the unhealthy food messages she got from her mother and father? "How to tell a teenager to try not to take it to heart?" she asks. "How do you tell someone to believe in themselves? I would just want to shake her and make it okay for her."

Your Family's Weight: What's at Stake

How does weight impact your family dynamic? The answers to this question go far beyond the number on the scale, as research has shown us.

Your sex life: Interestingly, science suggests that weight can have a measurable effect on the quality of the marital relationship. In a 2011 study in the *Journal of Sex and Marital Therapy*, Duke University researchers found that obesity has a detrimental effect on sexual quality of life between couples.[5] And it doesn't take a scientist to tell us how a downturn in intimacy can affect other parts of your relationship with your spouse.

Your children's long-term health: Many other studies have found clear connections between the weight status of parents and that of their children. In 2012, Stamatis Efstathiou, MD, MSc, PhD, and colleagues studied Greek households and determined that home and family environment—particularly involving diet and activity choices—appears likely to be a very strong predictor of childhood obesity.[6] Professional organizations are taking notice, and in 2012 the American Heart Association issued a scientific statement calling parents and other adult caregivers "agents of change" for their obese children, based on a review of existing literature. The AHA researchers found that parents who instituted changes to encourage behaviors associated with healthier weight in the home environment tended to be more successful in affecting the weight of their children.

Your family's emotional well-being: The picture emerging from a number of studies[7,8,9] shows that our weight and the weight of those to whom we are related are associated with levels of stress and depression within the family. While other factors may be involved, researchers suggest that the connection here is more than just coincidence—evidenced by a 2013 study in the *Journal of Epidemiology and Public Health* in which Spanish researchers showed obesity in childhood and adolescence to be an independent risk factor for depression in adult life.[10]

Miriam knows she cannot go back in time, but she can correct the negative messages of the past for her own children.

"That's one thing with my kids I always do. I tell them they're good enough," she says.

And after a thoughtful pause, she adds, "I may have gone overboard. They think they're too good."

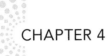

How Your Friends Can Make—Or Break— Your Weight Success

Aside from your actual relatives, your friends are probably the people you "relate" to most. After all, as much as you may love them, you don't choose most members of your family. When it comes to your likes, your dislikes, and the way you spend your time away from home and work, these individuals are most likely to mirror your personal choices.

So to butcher a metaphor—if your friends are the proverbial birds, your thoughts and actions are the familiar feathers. You are all covered in them as you flock together to the movies, to the restaurant, to the wine and cheese party at your best friend's house.

All of this begs the question: Are those "feathers" making you fat?

Now that we've adequately tortured this turn of phrase, let's look at the story of a woman whose relationships with friends and acquaintances contributed to her weight gain and see how a change in her social circle outside of her home made all the difference.

This is the story of Marcia, a former patient of Malissa. At sixty-two years old, she had struggled with obesity since her twenties. Part of this had to do with habits and routines she had followed as far back as she could remember. She had always had trouble controlling the strong

connection she felt between her brain and her stomach. Eating carbs made her feel good, plain and simple. But these positive feelings had a negative side, both for her weight and her health. At her heaviest, Marcia weighed 308 pounds. She was on five blood pressure medications, but her blood pressure would still spike on occasion, sometimes reaching 210/150. A normal blood pressure, by comparison, is 120/80 or less. In short, it was a dangerous situation.

Looking back, it was easy for Marcia to see how day-to-day demands took a toll on her social life. A clinical psychologist with a doctorate in psychology, Marcia was also a parent, raising three stepsons, and she was a caregiver for her aging mother. These were rewarding endeavors, but they meant she was often too busy to cultivate new friendships and had very little time for her existing ones. Instead of coping with the pressures of her busy life by talking with friends, she turned to food for comfort. The few friends she had were not living particularly healthy lifestyles, either. Marcia admits that the close friends with whom she spent the most time outside of home and work were all "a little bit heavyset." No one in her social circle exercised or made real efforts to eat a healthy diet, and while she and her friends would often lament about their unhealthy weight, none within her social circle ever did much about the problem. Marcia would sometimes attempt to make her routine healthier, but while her friends were supportive in other aspects of her life, they remained out of step with these occasional efforts. Soon enough, she would always return to her typical diet and sedentary lifestyle.

Marcia knew she had to take action, though, when one day, alone at home, she fell and could not get up. She had to call the fire department for help.

By this time, Marcia had only one child living at home, a teenage daughter who was also battling the scale. When Marcia finally made an appointment to see Malissa, she was desperate for change, both for herself and for her daughter. That's when Malissa recommended she join a group program built around exercise, healthy eating, and positive support called Learn to Be Lean, led by the Cardiovascular Disease Prevention Center at Massachusetts General Hospital.

For Marcia, joining the group was more powerful than any prescription. It literally gave her an emergency dose of friendship. For the first time in her life, she was surrounded by people who shared a similar interest in improving their health. And Marcia's new habits had a spillover effect. At home, she and her daughter made an all-out assault on the pantry—throwing away processed, high-sugar, high-carb foods and replacing them with minimally processed foods, as well as an abundance of fresh fruits and vegetables.

It was an adjustment at first. Marcia was challenged by her new exercise and diet regimen. But she quickly recognized something different about this particular weight loss attempt: The support she got from her new friends was motivating and invaluable. For the first time in many years, Marcia was surrounded by people who actually cared about her life and her journey toward health. They made her feel that she was a part of a circle of friends who shared a common goal. She found the positive atmosphere in the group almost addictive. By the end of the three-month program, Marcia had begun to see her weight come off—and, more important, she had made lifestyle changes that made weight loss seem less of a hurdle. Convinced that the social connection was the deciding factor in her success, she went in search of another network of like-minded people and found a regular water aerobics class at her nearby YMCA.

While she maintained her relationships with her old, dear friends, the interactions Marcia had with her new, healthy friends extended outside of the classes. Some of these women, in fact, had been Marcia's acquaintances from work; they now enjoyed a closer familiarity, kindled by their exercise classes.

Over two years, Marcia's perseverance led to a weight loss of more than 130 pounds. Her general health improved as well. Before, she had to take "a bag of pills every day" to deal with the health issues brought about by her weight. As the weight came off, though, her doctor gradually reduced the number of medications she needed, and she got down to one prescription pill a day.

Technically speaking, Marcia's transformation was the result of diet and exercise. However, there's no doubt in her mind that the best medicine was really her new group of friends.

A Little Help from Your Friends

If there were a shopping mall that sold the full range of actions we could take to live a healthier life, motivation would be the money in our wallets. Whether from a book, the people around us, or our own internal voice, motivation is the currency we spend to make ourselves exercise or eat more responsibly. We can use it to do the things we might actually prefer not to do—or at least the things we think we don't want to do at first. And our friends can be a powerful source of motivation for us if we let them.

In Marcia's previous attempts at weight loss, she relied on her own motivation. It was strong enough to get her through the first few workouts and the first week or so of healthy eating. But within a few weeks, or even days, her resolve would give way, and she would slip back into old patterns. Only when she was surrounded by people who had the healthy habits she was trying to develop did her motivation increase. For Marcia, this happened during group exercise sessions in the pool. "I was happy that there were forty people in the water with me," Marcia says. "I felt happy to be moving to the beat of music. I went from absolutely not liking exercise to loving it—the positive reinforcement was the key to my success."

Granted, our relationship with our friends is not the first thing that comes to mind for most of us when we look at the numbers on the scale. But in reality a fair amount of research has been devoted to determining the effect friendship has on exercise and other behaviors that affect our health and weight. As it turns out, simply having a strong social network—no matter what you and your friends like to do together—is a plus for your health.

Let's start with the most basic indicator of health—in a word, survival. Lisa Berkman, PhD, of Harvard University conducted a seminal study in this area in 1979 involving more than seven thousand adults.[1]

She found that those who had the fewest or least supportive relationships tended to die younger than those who were more involved with their friends and within their communities. It sounds mysterious, but the reason why is pretty simple: People who have many friends or even just a few close friendships are more likely to take care of themselves. At a minimum, nearby friends are a bit like a surrogate family; they can remind us to attend doctor appointments and take our medicines or can provide transportation to grocery stores or clinics, especially when we are not feeling well. Friendships also make a difference in the outcome when we do become seriously ill. In a study that Walter was involved with, led by Harvard's Ichiro Kawachi, MD, PhD, simply being part of a tightly knit social network didn't predict whether someone was obese or whether they would have a heart attack in the future. But those with more extensive social networks—both in terms of quantity of contacts and the quality of these relationships—were less likely to die if they did have a heart attack.[2]

Some of this research—even through focusing primarily on survival—also begins to show how lacking such connections could be linked to behaviors that have unfortunate effects on our weight. University of Arizona behavioral scientist Chris Segrin, PhD, discovered that people who define themselves as lonely consume more alcohol, eat foods higher in unhealthy fat, and exercise less than those who report being more socially connected.[3] Other researchers through various works have reinforced this finding. Scottish researchers, for example, have pointed to a link between a lackluster social life and such factors as smoking and obesity.[4] They also reported a specific lack of desire among lonely people to lose weight through exercise.

What does all of this tell us? Sharing our experiences with other people helps to buffer us against many behaviors that are very obviously harmful to our health, weight, and well-being. And friends—the right kind of friends, anyway—are likely to encourage us when we take steps that clearly improve our weight and how we see ourselves. So not only can the support and friendship of a group soften the blow of giving up problem overeating or drinking, it also provides a cheering section when your waistline shrinks six inches!

Of course, as we suggested, this happens when you have the *right* kind of friends. What most of us know from intuition or past experience is that simply having connections does not always guarantee that we will be healthier. Take the results from a Harvard-led study published in the journal *Preventive Medicine*[5] as an example: People who had the highest level of social support—in other words, those who felt they would be able to get help from those they knew if they needed it—reported the highest fruit and vegetable intake, as well as more exercise. But not so fast. These highly sociable people also reported eating more red meat and junk food. Translation: It wouldn't be unusual if your walking buddy was the same person you meet for beers and pizza with extra cheese and pepperoni. Thus, while a strong social network is, in general, desirable, it can have both positive and negative influences that are important to understand.

Here's a fun way to visualize these positive and negative influences in our relationships with our friends. If you were a kid in the 1970s or 1980s, or perhaps even a parent of a kid at this time, think back to the time when playgrounds were not the wood-chipped, plastic monuments to safety that they are today. Among the rusted metal attractions (some today might call them death traps) on which kids whiled away their hours, there was often a piece of equipment that resembled sort of a four-way seesaw. The suggested method of play was clear—four seats for four kids, each trying to out-bounce the other three.

But things got really fun when a fifth person made the bold (and in retrospect, unsafe) decision to test their balance by standing on the hub in the middle of these four arms—and, a bit like a surfer riding a wave, seeing how many seconds they could remain standing before falling toward one direction or the other.

There is a fitting metaphor here for the influence you get from your friends. Like the kid standing in the middle of the four-way seesaw, we are all subject to the weight influences of the friends with whom we interact. As any individual tilts the balance their way, so do we feel ourselves sliding one way or the other—except in this case, the direction we slide has implications for our weight.

But you, unlike the kid in the middle of the seesaw, actually have some control over the way your friends influence your weight You can learn to tease out the negative influences and reinforce the positive ones. Malissa and her colleagues demonstrated this in one aspect of the HAPPY Heart study. They brought obese women who were socially isolated together to meet regularly, talk about healthy eating, and take exercise classes. Over a two-year period, the women were able to incorporate regular physical activity and better nutrition into their lives. The women were empowered with information provided through group sessions where they learned and discussed the nuts and bolts of nutrition. They learned how to read labels and ways of minimizing sugars and saturated fats in their diet. And, most important, they used this knowledge to influence the individual choices that were made within their social group. The women went on group grocery-shopping trips and learned how to shop the perimeter of the store to find low-cost, fresher foods and to avoid the middle aisles stocked with sodium- and calorie-laden snack foods. They shared recipes with one another and learned how to create healthy meals on a budget for their families. They shared their experiences of trying to cook for teenagers, picky husbands, and in-laws. They worked together with the nutritionist to modify favorite family recipes. In short, they piled onto the healthy side of the seesaw for each other, making it much more likely that everyone would tumble toward a healthier weight.

Later in this chapter, we will get into the specifics of programs like HAPPY Heart in terms of the weight loss and improvements in health these women enjoyed. But for now, it's important to see that the evidence from programs like Learn to Be Lean and results from the HAPPY Heart study affirm that having friends who practice healthy behaviors will tilt you toward health, too—and we can infer from this that being surrounded by people with unhealthy behaviors can likewise lead you in that direction. What your friends do greatly determines what you eat, whether you exercise, and ultimately what you weigh.

Why You Don't Have to Choose between Your Friends and Your Weight

Which interactions with our friends actually help us achieve our weight goals, and which hurt us? As it turns out, it comes down to the combination of the situation we are in and the friends who are with us at the time.

Think about the time you spend with your friends. What do you do

How Hidden Social Cues Can Play a Part in Weight Gain

The influences that make us eat more or exercise less without our noticing speak to the often-hidden tendency of others' behavior to affect our own. The impact is often subtle, and your reaction to it may be unconscious, but it definitely is there.

Take, for example, a study conducted by Dutch researchers[6] in which they paired 140 young women for a meal to examine their eating habits as they sat across from each other. While these women enjoyed their food and conversation, the researchers meticulously counted the number of bites that each woman took of her meal. When they compared the number of bites, they found not only that it was very similar for each woman, but also that the rate at which the women ate their meals was similar over the course of their encounter. This mimicking could be a good thing if either woman was being mindful of what she was doing and how rapidly her fork completed the circuit between her plate and her mouth. But it also means that if one of these women overeats, her lunch companion might very well overeat, too—a simple social interaction together and what do you talk about? Particularly if you happen to be a woman, it's pretty likely that weight issues and health habits tend to creep into your usual conversation. And, let's be honest, most of the time the tone is negative. Try to remember the last time you heard this from someone in your social circle: "My problem is that I just have too much time to exercise and plan out healthy meals."

Exactly. We couldn't either.

Complaining to our friends, particularly when we feel guilty about not meeting our obligations to ourselves in terms of exercise or diet, is practically a reflex. And when your friends commiserate and share their

that could have a surprising amount of influence.

Also demonstrating how social situations can interact with our personalities to lead to unhealthy weight behaviors, a team of researchers used a questionnaire to identify individuals who were "people pleasers."[7] You know these people. You may even be one of them. If this is the case, you can indeed empathize with their strong desire to maintain harmony in social gatherings. But this study showed that you might be doing them a huge favor by not offering them that bowl of unhealthy snacks. The researchers found that people pleasers tended to eat more of the food they were offered—whether they were actually hungry for it or not. These study subjects, it turned out, were simply reacting to a situation where social eating was "expected" in terms of conforming to the norm. And it doesn't take too many of these gatherings before their waistlines start paying the price.

The thing is, these social situations are not at all uncommon. The same factors pervade the most common encounters we have with our friends—heading out to grab a bite to eat or meeting at a friend's apartment for a birthday celebration. When we are with our friends, whether we are conscious of it or not, we are constantly receiving and transmitting cues that indicate the expected norm. And we might be having such a good time that we don't even realize what is happening on our plates and forks, or in our mouths.

own difficulties, you naturally feel it is more acceptable to just maintain the status quo. This status quo for many, unfortunately, involves inactivity and a sugar- and carb-packed, "more convenient" diet.

These discussions, along with unspoken but observed behaviors like the lunch meetings that always seem to include dessert and the covert agreements to skip your afternoon jog "just this once" to take a trip to the mall, surreptitiously support and reinforce bad choices.

Clearly the solution is for each of us to determine how our social situations will inevitably affect our diet and other lifestyle choices. In reality, it is so much more comfortable to be surrounded by others who share our own values. After all, it is odd to see an avid amateur athlete surrounded by sedentary, obese friends. And it makes sense that choosing to spend time with friends who reinforce healthy choices rather than unhealthy ones can go a long way in terms of tilting the field in your favor when it comes to your weight. But, as we have discussed, we also know that the opposite is true. And if we are really being honest with ourselves, we already know that we may enjoy our time spent within a variety of our social circles in which behaviors and routines related to diet and exercise are not as friendly to your waistline or overall health as they should be.

Does this mean that you will need to abandon your social circle to lose weight? Fortunately, in most cases it does not. And here's why.

Think for a moment about all of the interactions you have with your friends. Some focus explicitly on food—going out to dinner and dessert, for example. Others potentially have little to do with food at all—going shopping, heading to a museum, or taking in a concert. And then there are others that, at first glance, seem to have little to do with eating, but during which some unhealthy options can creep in. After all, for some people a trip to the movies just isn't complete without that colossal tub of buttered popcorn.

If you happen to be friends with someone who is an unhealthy influence whenever tempting food creeps into your activities, maybe this is not the best person to be around during certain activities. But that doesn't mean you have to cut them out of your life. There are probably ways you can change up the activity or venue—mini golf or bowling instead of dinner, or maybe even a physical activity you both enjoy so much, you don't even realize you are doing something healthy at the same time!

This means you might end up with more opportunities to enjoy the social events that do involve food with your friends who practice more healthy food habits. So while you've probably heard about "division of labor," what we're talking about here is a "division of leisure"—saving your stomach for that friend of yours who is more likely to introduce you to a tasty and healthy new way to cook a fish for dinner, and shifting away from potential land mines by changing the venue on your less-healthy friends. You can also block out the time you consider prime for physical activity with those friends who actually engage in enjoyable exercise, and meet with your less-active friends during times you would not be exercising anyway. You may even find that you can take the best elements of your healthy interactions and apply them to get-togethers with other people in your social circle. Before long you may be preparing healthy dinners with the same friends who, weeks before, had encouraged you to polish off a platter of hot wings. Or perhaps you can share some fun and healthful outdoor activities that you discovered from other acquaintances. Who knows? One or more of your friends could be ready for a change that will help them shift into a healthier lifestyle as well.

The bottom line: It makes sense to handpick a set of friends who will support your choices in the early phase of making healthy changes in your life. Tap into the Thinfluential ability of your friends whose health habits you would hope to share. Again, this doesn't mean you have to dump your friends who don't necessarily share your new approach to managing your weight; it just means you need to spend less time with them until your new approach to eating, drinking, and exercising is ingrained. When you reach that point, you are ready to become the Thinfluencer in their lives.

Getting Organized:
The Power of Groups

We've spent a lot of time talking about separating the friends who encourage you to adopt healthy behaviors from those who cause you to lean toward unhealthy behaviors. But what if having friends on both sides of this fence is not your situation?

You may find after some consideration that you actually have few to no friends who practice healthy weight behaviors. Or perhaps you have so

Finding the Most Influential Friends in Your Network

Whether we have few friends or many, the sheer size of our social networks, once we add in various degrees of separation, is probably far greater than we realize. We are connected to a wide variety of people—some who happen to be more influential than others, some who are more susceptible to outside influence. This, too, has been studied in detail,[8,9] in many cases using data provided through social media like Facebook—mainly since this information is so widely available and measures the actions of millions of people. Researchers have also used more traditional methods of studying social networks. The important thing to be aware of, though, is that within any extended social group, some people's actions are more likely to be impactful to the group than those of others.

This is what a team of researchers from three institutions in Colorado reported in a 2009 study in the journal *Obesity*.[10] When they analyzed the way that obesity spread through social networks, they found that focusing efforts on certain well-connected individuals may be the best strategy for breaking the cycle of obesity within a social network.

When we look more closely at

few close friends that it would be difficult or impossible to apply the strategies discussed.

That's okay! This is where organized group activities come in. Even if you find yourself alone in your desire to take action, options in your community may allow you to join a ready-made social circle formed around healthy behaviors.

The advantage to joining a group focused on healthy lifestyle choices is that you will not have to negotiate with your friends to adopt healthier behaviors—a tricky situation, particularly if you have just recently begun efforts to achieve a healthier weight. Such groups are available in most

these dynamics, some very interesting trends start to emerge. We see, for example, that while simply having friends who are not obese may help buoy your efforts, it's when your *friends'* friends are in shape and enjoy a healthy weight that you reap an even greater positive effect.

With this realization, we see our social connections are more than just individual threads—they start to weave themselves into a tapestry. And like any tapestry, the fabric at the edges is more likely to fray.

So to return to the topic of this section of the chapter—the trick might not be to cut off your relationships with those who have unhealthy habits, nor is it to simply forge stronger bonds with those who live at a healthy weight. Rather, it may be to find the connections who are most ensconced within the fabric of healthy habits and actions—in other words, those who are healthy and whose friends and acquaintances are also healthy.

Likewise, even aiming to strengthen connections with those who are not necessarily at their healthiest weight, but who are nested among those who practice healthy lifestyles, may be a good move. Strengthening these connections may be beneficial not only for you, but also for this individual who is dissatisfied with her weight yet still near the center of a healthy social tapestry. Your efforts to strengthen such a bond could be just the thing to "tighten the stitches" for both of you, leading to weight and lifestyle changes that are more likely to endure.

communities, and given the usual range of options, a little bit of reconnaissance work can often go a long way toward finding groups in your area that can help you along, especially if it's hard to get yourself motivated to make a change.

One of the most popular options is Weight Watchers, which has franchises in communities around the world and even features an online community for those who do not live close to one of their centers. This program is not the only option—numerous hospitals and other medical and commercial institutions offer them as well. But, if you find that a Weight Watchers program is your cup of tea, you'll probably be glad to know that a number of studies have examined this group approach, and it appears to be an effective solution for many people.[11,12,13] In perhaps one of the largest of these studies,[14] British researchers evaluated nearly thirty thousand overweight and obese people who had been referred to the Weight Watchers program by their doctors. Of those who actually completed the first course of the program, more than half lost 5 percent or more of their body weight.

But is a group approach like this really more effective than simply going it alone? Again, studies suggest that the answer to this question is a resounding yes. Research presented at the 2010 International Congress on Obesity[15] specifically compared overweight and obese adults participating in Weight Watchers to those who chose the solo route instead. The results? Participants in the lifestyle modification group lost about twice as much weight over the year as those who went solo. This finding actually falls well into line with the overall philosophy and psychology of group efforts, which has long emphasized that groups are more than just the sum of their parts. While each member can accomplish a little, the power of the collective group far exceeds that of the individual.

So the researchers' message here makes perfect sense: A group approach—in fact, any group approach—can empower individuals to accomplish what they couldn't accomplish alone. It is far more than peer pressure; others can demonstrate how to go about making changes and can share their struggles and successes.

Malissa's HAPPY Heart study, too, is a great example of what can be accomplished in a group setting as far as behaviors that shape your weight. By sharing their personal experiences, the women developed a deeper bond with their peers. A key advantage of working together was the ability of the group to focus not only on the solution but also on the obstacles in their lives that led them to make poor choices on a daily basis. The group recognized and discussed the idea that it is all about habits: Once something becomes ingrained in the fabric of your life, it becomes tolerable at first, then acceptable, and, finally, comfortable. This goes for adoption of new ways of eating and exercising as well as for unhealthy habits like avoidance of exercise and poor nutrition. The difference is in your frame of reference.

This new network of social support coupled with information had a profound impact on the women's overall health. The women ate out less, skipped fewer meals, and ate diets lower in calories and processed sugars and higher in fruits and vegetables. They started practicing portion control. The women were also more likely to incorporate regular exercise into their daily lives and looked forward to walking together and going to Zumba, yoga, and relaxation classes with their new friends. These changes in behavior translated into tangible health benefits.

They also managed to lose weight around their middles (and keep it off), and their blood sugar and blood pressures dropped significantly. The average waist measurement decreased from 41.5 inches to 38.6 inches. Their average systolic blood pressures dropped seven points, a very significant change. Their HDL "good" cholesterol numbers increased, on average, from 44.5 to 49.3, and their glucose levels improved as well. These positive changes correlated with simultaneous reductions in measures of stress, depression, and anxiety—psychological factors we know can wreak havoc on our health if they aren't controlled and certainly undermine attempts at positive behavior changes. This study demonstrated that even those lacking a social support system can create this network by reaching out to those who share similar obstacles to good health in their daily lives. They would reach out to one another to help handle the daily challenges they had not successfully managed before. They learned to laugh with one another (laughter yoga was a favorite group activity) and reached out to support those who came upon tough times.

Does your group have to be a formally established program like this one? Not necessarily. What is important is having a set time, location, and regimen—three crucial ingredients when establishing a new norm within your group of friends. And unlike so many of the other norms to which you may be accustomed, these will be built around healthy behaviors like regular exercise and smart diet habits.

But if the idea of an organized lifestyle modification group appeals to you, ask around or go online and research what is available in your area. Some places that are likely to offer these services may include medical institutions, the local Y, or possibly commercial franchises. As you get more information about such programs, you may learn that this approach is worth a shot for your goals. Several national Web sites are also dedicated to connecting people with interest in similar activities such as walking (such as walkingconnection.com), hiking (check out www.comehike.com), or cycling (try the Adventure Cycling Association, at www.adventurecycling.org). Even if you don't have friends in your close circle who are taking on a new healthy habit, you can certainly look for and find them in your community.

Thinfluence Action Plan: Your Social Circle

By now you have probably already begun to reflect on some of the common interactions in your own social circles that help or hinder your weight-related efforts based on the information earlier in this chapter. Through the Thinfluence Action Plan exercise below, you will be able to put together some solutions that will help you deal with the situations that regularly arise when you are among your friends.

ANALYZE

1. How do you spend your time when interacting with your social circle?

A. Whether dinner, lunch, or drinks, food is almost always the centerpiece of the occasion. And physical activity? Forget about it!

B. It's about an even split between indulgence and activity. Sure, we have the occasional tasty treat or cocktail, but we walk and exercise together on occasion as well.

C. Whether engaging in a regular walk, hiking a trail, or playing a pickup game of tennis, my friends and I are usually on the move. Healthy snacks and a cool glass of water, please!

2. Think of your closest friends—those with whom you spend the most time. Would you say these relationships are:

A. Detrimental to my health and weight, if I had to answer honestly. Few, if any, of the activities we do together are healthy.

B. Neutral to my health and weight. I don't necessarily feel that my friends are keeping me from achieving and maintaining a healthy weight, but I don't feel as if they are encouraging me in my efforts either.

C. Conducive to improvements in my health and weight. I have to admit that my friends seem even more enthused about a healthy weight than I am sometimes. I find their attitude infectious.

3. What do you think would happen if you suggested starting a healthy new routine (or ending an unhealthy one) among your social circle?

A. I don't think my friends would be open to changing their routines.

B. My friends would probably get on board with healthy changes if I brought the issue up.

C. I think it would be easy to get my friends involved in healthy new ideas.

ACT

Take a look at your answers to these three questions. Where do your responses fall?

◊ Mostly As: You're not alone. This is probably where many people are, and it's not the easiest starting point for change. However, this tells you that finding an organized weight loss group may be the right strategy for you—particularly if you are just starting your efforts to improve your weight. Remember, this group approach can be anything from a lifestyle modification group offered by a medical institution or local franchise to a community sports league. Once you find one that works for you, stick with it. You'll see results.

◊ Mostly Bs: Not too bad! It sounds like your friends may be receptive to your ideas for a new norm within your group, one that incorporates more healthy behaviors and eliminates the unhealthy ones. See what steps you can take to change the nature of your socializing from less "intake-based" activities—eating, sitting while watching entertainment—to a more output-based, dynamic model. This could involve exercise or other activities that involve "doing" rather than "taking in." Maybe yoga, walking in a public garden, hiking, or riding bicycles. Get creative!

◊ Mostly Cs: If you are in this situation, congratulations—it is a rare and ideal spot to be in. Chances are, if you can answer C for all of the questions above, strong norms are already in place within your group. So the question you should be asking yourself is: Are you taking full advantage of this great influence from your social circle? Recognize that there is always room for improvement. Sometimes it makes sense to switch up a shared routine to keep the momentum going. Mix it up. Instead of the same old run, pull that bike down from the rafters, pump up the tires, and go on a group ride this weekend. Activities like biking and hiking certainly lend themselves not only to nurturing our health, but also to strengthening our friendships.

Make a short list (it will be a short one indeed!) of friends you know will support you completely as you strive to make some changes. Think of ways to spend a bit more time with them over the next few months.

Make another list (likely longer) of those friends who are comfortable

Your Emergency Exits

Hors d'oeuvre–heavy holiday parties. Alcohol-focused get-togethers with friends. So many social situations entail high-calorie indulgences, you may feel as if the deck is regularly stacked against you.

In these situations, simply saying no may feel as if you are committing a faux pas—and may be met by such responses as "Jane thought you loved her pecan pie!" or "It's one drink! Why don't you toast with us anymore?"

If you are on the straight and narrow in your diet, it's tough to be surrounded by people who are indulging. The trick is to be prepared. It's good to go in with a list of scripts you can use as your "emergency exits" from these social obligations. Here are a few that might work for you:

◊ "These hors d'oeuvres are too good! I am cutting myself off to save room for the lovely dinner!"

◊ "That looks fantastic! Unfortunately, my doctor won't let me have that. Sad but true!"

◊ "I would love to have a drink, but I have to go back into work later. Have to stay sharp!"

Come up with your own and practice them until you are comfortable with them. If you go into potentially problematic situations with a game plan, you may be surprised to find how easy it is to make healthier choices.

The "Nudge Factor"—
How to Be Persistent, Not Pushy

The nudge factor is a major consideration when dealing with friends and other valued relationships. After all, the line between encouragement and alienation can sometimes be thin. Below are a few tips that may help you approach your friends with suggestions for how to incorporate healthy habits into their regular routines, without seeming too pushy.

Lead by example: So often we hear the phrase "Actions speak louder than words." Be patient and focus on yourself and your own actions first. As you become more mindful of how you adjust to take on the unhealthy norms within your social group, you will begin to learn how to avoid them and improve your own habits. Once your friends see the results of your lifestyle changes, trust us, they'll be asking you for advice!

Start with a few small adjustments, but stick to these resolutions: Remember when we told you in Chapter 1 that if you can do just one small thing to start, it can provide the momentum you need to get on a healthier lifestyle path? The same principle applies to those in your social circle. Don't try to encourage someone close to you to completely overhaul their life; they'll be less likely to adopt these changes, and the chances that they will misinterpret your actions as judgmental are high. Instead, try starting small. Introduce a minor change to your usual routine—for example, meeting at a new deli instead of the cupcake shop where you always meet. If she asks, tell your friend that you made the change to satisfy your own curiosity or that you had heard good things about the place. If you frame your healthy choices as things you are doing for yourself rather than as suggestions or direct advice, you will be offering your friend the chance to take her own initiative.

Push less, praise more: If you get a friend or two to do something healthy for themselves, be ready to encourage them. Whenever you can, point out the progress they have made. Focusing on what they are doing right, rather than what they still need to improve, puts a positive spin on your influence, which is likely to give them incentive to keep on the right track.

with the status quo and who you think actually like spending time with you because you support or endorse their unhealthy choices. Take a little break from spending lots of time with them—for now! Nothing is more likely to shoot down your efforts at avoiding that big plate of nachos than hanging out with the group you typically meet for Mexican food and margaritas.

INFLUENCE

Now that you have a strategy, see if you can formulate some selling points you can use both to convince others around you to join you in your efforts and to strengthen your own resolve to stick with your plan. Create a list of the goals and incentives that are a driving force behind your change. What might these look like?

Goal: Better weight control for both you and your friends

Incentive: Improved quality of life and health, more energy, lowered blood pressure and body mass index, fewer trips to the doctor—not to mention you will look better in your clothes!

Goal: A broadened base of fun activities for your social circle to enjoy together

Incentive: Closer friendships nurtured by frequent, healthy interactions

Goal: A fresh approach to leisure time that opens your social circle up to healthful activities and experiences

Incentive: Potential for new relationships, opening the door to new, healthier routines

These possibilities should motivate you to take that first step—followed by the next step and the next step after that—toward your goal.

Are You Ready to Walk?

Forming a group to do something as simple as walking can have big dividends for your health, weight, and well-being. For those who participate, the feeling of being part of a group can be a strong motivation—after all, if the group activity occurs on a certain time and day, your group will wonder where you are if you are not there! This positive influence will significantly improve the chances you will follow through with your exercise. Plus, it gives you the chance to positively influence others. Imagine the inspiration you will pass on to others in the neighborhood as they see your healthy group walking by!

Here are a few tips to help you get started.

If you want to start a walking group but you live in a rural area that is not walking-friendly: Think about establishing a community walking path. Walter cleared out just such a walking path near his family's cabin in New Hampshire, cutting through the grass and brush to create a safe route for a pleasant hike. In fact, his family's interest in such a trail got other people in the community's conservation committee involved in its construction—a perfect example of the Thinfluence ripple effect. Those involved in developing the path are more likely to use it. A relatively small investment of time turned into a healthy resource for the entire community.

If you live in an urban area where you or some of your friends feel unsafe: This is where it becomes important to invoke the "safety in numbers" rule. Through her programs, Malissa was able to create walking groups among women who lived in urban areas that would meet up on Saturday and Wednesday mornings—times that were not only convenient for those involved, but also safe times of day in their neighborhoods. Additionally, being in a group contributed to the feeling of safety.

If you're having trouble finding enough people to join you: Try tapping the power of social media! The community aspects of social media platforms like Facebook, as well as shared blogs and bulletin boards, can all be important tools for establishing a network of people who may be interested in joining a fitness group. Start a Facebook page devoted to your weekly walking outings—invitation-only, just for your walking group. Use this as a home base for setting meeting times, tips, and encouragement.

You may wish to choose simple strategies that you can apply easily and immediately to get yourself started. Remember: You don't have to do everything at once. Examine your routines with your friends and acquaintances and identify the behaviors that undermine your weight and health. Pick one and work on it; when you have made headway, move down the list. Even applying just one or two of the strategies you come up with to your social life may go a long way toward a healthier weight for you as well as for your friends.

A Helping Hand Up, Back on the Wagon

One more thing about Marcia's story illustrates the power of friendships when it comes to weight control. Months after she achieved her 130-pound weight loss, she found herself returning to old habits. Before long, she had regained some of the weight she had lost. But she had a safety net that caught her before she slipped all the way back to her old weight.

It wasn't a crash diet or a surgery or an extreme exercise boot camp. She simply remembered what it felt like to be healthy. And then she packed up her gym bag and went back to the friends she had made in her water-aerobics class.

"I was cheered by everybody," Marcia says. "They welcomed me with open arms. They told me: 'You can do it, Marcia. You did it once before. You can do it again.'"

After being back in her healthier routine for a few months, Marcia lost ten of the thirty pounds she had put back on. Now she has her sights set on her target weight of 170 pounds.

What Marcia's story shows is that making lifestyle changes, however subtle, can be tough. Falling off the wagon, losing track of a routine, slacking off at the gym, or indulging inappropriately at the dinner table are easy mistakes to make. While the members of the group may have different individual goals, the common goal of improving and then maintaining their exercise and nutrition habits helps keep the momentum going. Life's little obstacles are unavoidable; it is resilience to these and the support of friends that helps us get back on track. The accountability provided by a group cannot be overestimated. Knowing that your friends will be checking in on you if you miss a workout is a good motivator to push you out of bed in the morning.

And this is precisely what makes our friends and social groups so important. The emotional support that one receives from a team of friends

Making It Stick

Getting your friends to join you in your weight-slashing aspirations may seem daunting at first, but you can do many simple things to make it easier for you and your friends to start a group for healthy activities.

Make it cheap: If you want to get a group of friends together to exercise regularly, be mindful of the costs. The less expensive you make it, the more people can join you and the more likely it is that people will stick with the group. Walking around your neighborhood or a local school's track is obviously free, save for the cost of a pair of walking shoes. But you could do other budget-minded activities together.

For instance, start a strength-training group. Members could meet at each other's homes twice a week. You can all work out to an exercise video or do a workout you found in a book or magazine. Many strength-training routines rely on just your body weight—think squats, lunges, pushups, and crunches. But for a minor investment ($9 to $12), you each could purchase an exercise band. These multipurpose rubber bands offer all of the workout possibilities of a set of dumbbells. To perform biceps curls, loop one end around your toes and use the other end as you would any other weight, curling up and down in slow, like this cannot be underestimated. Social groups and friendships let us share our routines and healthy lifestyle tips, but they are also there for us to share our successes, our failures, and our desire to improve.

However, for many of us, other social interactions may have just as great—or perhaps even greater—an influence over our day-to-day choices and actions. These interactions take place at the workplace, where many of us spend a significant portion of our waking hours. In the next chapter, we will see the various ways in which the work environment plays a part in your weight.

controlled movements. For a triceps workout, wrap the band around your back, hold one end of the loop in each fist, and slowly punch in front of you, left followed by right. Best of all, these bands take up virtually no space—you can even carry them in your pocket.

And what if you want to apply the same sort of economic reasoning to healthy eating habits? You could replace a regular outing to a calorie-heavy dinner on the town with an evening in with your friends, preparing your own food. Not only does this satisfy the penny-pincher in all of us, but it also gives us far more control over what we are eating.

Make it easy (and convenient): If you imagine that you'll get your friends out of bed at 5:00 a.m. to join you on a five-mile run four days a week, best of luck to you. Same goes for unrealistic and overly restrictive expectations for food choices. It's better to start with an activity or a healthy eating option that involves a convenient time and location and does not seem like a task. Make it easy for your friends to join you, and chances are your new routine will stick.

Make it fun: The most important part! You might even want to take advantage of preexisting routines. For example, if you have a regular poker night with your friends, make it an opportunity to serve healthy snacks instead of unhealthy ones. Or add a prize to your regular pot-luck: The healthiest and tastiest dish wins a prize. Nothing like some healthy competition!

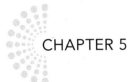

CHAPTER 5

Your Workplace
and Your Waistline

It is tempting to think of our problem with weight as a by-product of our choices during our leisure time. It is almost natural to believe that weight gain happens when we're sitting on the couch, watching television with a bag of chips in hand, or indulging in that second slice of cake after dinner. To think that it happens while we are in the middle of the workday hustle . . . well, that almost seems unfair.

But consider for a moment how most of your time is spent from day to day. A great percentage of us build our routines around our work schedule, and our workplaces are where many of us spend at least forty precious waking hours every week.

As much as we may hate to think about it (after all, don't we have enough to worry about at the office?), it is apparent that what we do at work plays an important role in our weight and health—at a time when balancing healthy and unhealthy behaviors may very well be the last thing on our minds.

This brings us to Jennifer, a fifty-five-year-old nurse and cardiac ultrasound technician working at Massachusetts General Hospital. Ironically, for someone whose work focused on making people healthy, Jennifer's life was anything but.

"The work that I did—working in a hospital—was tremendously

demanding," she recalls. "Meals were catch as catch can . . . . Let's just say it was hard to sit down and have a relaxing lunch, enjoy my food, and have any kind of rest time."

Nor was there much time for Jennifer to head outside for a quick break or walk. Her schedule was packed. Such was Jennifer's routine for ten hours a day, four days a week. Making matters worse, her commute added an hour and a half both in the morning and in the evening, which meant three more sedentary hours each day.

Away from work, Jennifer may have been able to mitigate the negative impacts of her work routine if she could unwind with some physical activity. But her time at home was largely spent in the role of caregiver for her mother, who was struggling with complications from both a heart attack and a stroke.

"It was a very stressful time, and I did not have a whole lot of time for myself," Jennifer says. "I was not exercising a lot, and being somewhat overweight and extremely overstressed, it only made things worse."

Ultimately her unforgiving routine showed up in the numbers—those on her scale, those describing her blood pressure and cholesterol scores, and the number of inches around her waist. At her unhealthiest point, Jennifer's five-foot-one-and-a-half frame weighed 179 pounds, and she was not even a bit surprised.

"You always hear people who say, 'I don't know why I'm overweight,'" Jennifer says. "Well, I know exactly why I was overweight. It was a lack of exercise. I eat healthy foods but big portions, and I tend to nibble a lot."

She had tried in the past to put the brakes on her weight gain, but to little avail. In these efforts, too, the pace and nature of her work were a formidable hurdle. She had signed up for gym memberships, only to find that her schedule prevented her from establishing a regular routine. "I transiently joined health clubs, only to end up 'giving them a donation' and not going there," she quips.

Jennifer knew she needed a change. Yet her situation appeared to present her with a stark decision: Should she stick with her current job and suffer the consequences to her weight and health? Or should she sacrifice her job to improve her health?

It's a choice that many of us—perhaps even most of us—may feel like we face from time to time. The good news is that the choice is false, which Jennifer found out at the beginning of 2012 when she joined the Be Fit program at Massachusetts General. This ten-week program focused on changes like getting at least thirty minutes of exercise five or more days a week and making healthy food choices. But one of the defining aspects of the program was the fact that it had different departments within the hospital engaged in a healthy competition with each other as they went through the program.

Working with Malissa, Jennifer began to make a series of small, simple, but important, changes to her work routine.

The first step she took was to change her workweek from four days to five; she cut her daily hours to eight. This little tweak gave her the opportunity to take different routes to work, which in turn allowed her some extra time in the mornings and evenings. Wisely, she used this time to start a walking routine. She started taking the elevator less and the stairs more. The fact that Jennifer's employer offered the Be Fit program was very convenient for her; she met once or twice a week with a personal trainer, who would go over her goals and progress with her. And while she admits that her eating habits did not change as much as they should have, the diary of eating and exercise habits she kept at least pointed her to potential areas of improvement.

But one of the most important changes occurred when Jennifer realized she was surrounded by colleagues who were involved in the program. These women became dependable allies in her weight and health battle.

"One of the girls in our department went through the program with tremendous changes in personal habits, weight loss, and a lot more physical activity," she says. "At that point I was much more motivated to try it."

When Jennifer couldn't make the meetings, her co-workers would catch her up on what she had missed. The team aspect of their progress was almost contagious.

"There's definitely a certain camaraderie," Jennifer says. "Many of the girls who did this were the front desk staff, who I know but did not know a whole lot. We got to talk a whole lot more about what we were doing, and that created a lot more support with some of the people."

In the ten weeks that Jennifer participated in the program, she lost ten pounds—a modest difference on the scale, but she says it allowed her to significantly change her body.

"I found I was actually enjoying exercise, and it had a significant improvement on my appearance," she says. "I definitely lost inches and toned up tremendously . . . . I saw my blood pressure come down significantly, and my LDL cholesterol went from 164 to 131.

"It was just very dramatic."

Your Workplace, Your Waistline

If you care at all about your job (as most of us do!), when you are at work, you are "in the zone." You might be concentrating too hard on the task at hand to realize how often you are snacking or how many hours pass by as you remain sedentary in your chair. You may not even notice how the workplace culture subtly reinforces the eating and activity patterns that you and your colleagues adopt. Yet as Jennifer's story demonstrates, the combination of these factors can hold tremendous sway over your weight.

Aside from being the place where we spend a great deal of our waking hours, the workplace is an important area for another reason, particularly if you happen to work in an office setting. In many ways, it is a microcosm in which so many of the dynamics in Thinfluence play a part. There is the social environment you share with your colleagues and acquaintances. There is the physical environment. Office and company policies come into play within the workplace. And myriad factors outside of the workplace, such as the surrounding neighborhood and available transportation options, affect how much time you spend going from home to work and back again each day.

In recent years, the central role that the workplace environment plays in our weight and health has been understood better, and these issues have attracted attention at the highest levels. In 2007, the World Health Organization, in conjunction with the World Economic Forum, organized a joint event to discuss their Global Strategy on Diet, Physical Activity and Health initiative—a strategy whose key elements include successful workplace health-promotion programs focusing on diet and physical activity. Specifically, the authors of the report noted:

> Workplaces are important settings for health promotion and disease prevention. People need to be given the opportunity to make healthy choices in the workplace in order to reduce their exposure to risk. Further, the cost to employers of morbidity attributed to noncommunicable diseases is increasing rapidly. Workplaces should make possible healthy food choices and support and encourage physical activity.[1]

As you can see from the Circles of Influence graph (page 10), we recognize the importance of the work environment by placing this circle just past your family and your friends. In other words, perhaps more than any of your surroundings, your workplace may be influencing your weight. The good news, of course, is that there are opportunities to make the positive factors in this environment work in your favor, while diminishing the effect of factors that are less than favorable to your waistline and health.

The Inactivity Problem

Whether you are a CEO, a telephone lineman, a homemaker, or a university professor, the fact that we all have different jobs—complete with different demands and expectations—is perhaps one of the most important reasons that there is no simple one-size-fits-all approach to healthy weight loss. Each of these jobs comes attached with its own "baseline" expectations of how much physical activity you will face in a normal day.

How much of a difference can the amount of baseline physical activity we get through our jobs make in our weight and health? As it turns out, quite a bit. The dramatic nature of this relationship has been represented in numerous studies; few, however, have drawn this connection more famously than a study by British epidemiologist Jerry Morris, conducted back in 1953, which compared heart attack rates between different workers who labored daily in the same environment—specifically, on double-decker buses.[2]

There are two very important jobs on a double-decker bus: a driver, obviously, to get the passengers where they need to go; and a conductor, who marches up and down the aisles to check the tickets. In Dr. Morris's study, the drivers and conductors were similar in almost every way—their socioeconomic status, the neighborhoods where they lived—except for the fact that their respective jobs had different sets of physical demands. The drivers remained seated for most of the day. The ticket-taking conductors, on the other hand, were on their feet, walking through the aisles of the bus and up and down between the upper and lower levels of the bus.

The longer these drivers and conductors held their jobs, the more different their bodies became. Dr. Morris verified this by tracking the trouser and jacket measurements for the conductors' uniforms and comparing them against the same measurements for the drivers' uniforms. It does not take much imagination to figure out who had the slimmer physiques in these duos. In addition, the drivers were nearly 50 percent more likely to have heart problems such as coronary artery disease.

So if you had to say that your job was more like that of the conductor or that of the driver, what would your answer be? If you happen to be employed as a Zumba instructor, or if you are an elite professional athlete, you will no doubt find that the requirements and environment of your job mean that you get more than enough physical activity to keep your weight and waistline under control. But if you are like the other 99.9 percent of the population, many of whom sit in front of a computer screen for hours on end, physical activity—and the opportunity to burn excess calories—could be a rare commodity indeed.

Because desk jobs have become so common in this day and age, the impact of sitting for extended periods at work is now of growing interest to researchers. At the forefront of this research is James Levine, MD, PhD, of Mayo Clinic, who for more than a decade has been studying how our workdays affect our obesity risk and health. Through a series of small studies, Dr. Levine has looked at the amount of time people spend sitting, standing, or walking during their workdays and their days off.[3,4,5] He has also meticulously quantified the differences in calories burned while engaged in all of these activities, all with the goal of figuring out the impact that sitting down for long periods potentially has on our waistlines.

If you happen to work at a desk job, you may find his conclusions disheartening. In a study in the journal *Obesity*, Dr. Levine found that subjects tended to sit for an additional one hundred minutes per day when at work.[6] These subjects also stood less and walked less while at work. Not surprisingly, the number of calories they burned each day through walking at work was about sixty calories lower than the calories burned while walking on the days they spent outside of the office. It may not seem like much at first, but day by day, the calorie total can add up, and end up, at your midsection.

The effect on our waistlines is only part of the problem, of course; a sedentary work routine has a much larger impact on our health than many may realize. As with the bus drivers, our hearts suffer. Heart disease is the number one killer of American men and women, and being inactive doubles your risk. The impacts extend to our weight status. Obesity is now widely considered to be the single most preventable cause of death among Americans.

Employers have big incentives to change the picture. Overweight and obesity are associated with decreased productivity, worsened health, and increased medical costs for employers. Unfortunately, obesity and inactivity are often nurtured in the workplace, most often in part due to the very nature of the jobs we perform.

Your Office Culture

Just as important as what you do at work are the people who surround you while you are there. Some of us refer to our colleagues as our "work family"— and just like family members, they are the ones whose behaviors and norms we tend to adopt. Sometimes this happens without our even knowing it, especially since while we are at work, the task at hand often seems more important than paying attention to actions that might be affecting our weight.

When Your Desk Is Your Gym

The sedentariness that many of us face daily at work has given rise to some interesting innovations in recent years. But few may be more interesting than the treadmill desk—an idea pioneered by the Mayo Clinic's James Levine, MD, PhD. As the name implies, the treadmill desk combines a treadmill and a desk. The result? Instead of sitting for eight hours a day while you work at your desk job, you will, at the very least, be standing and probably walking.

Dr. Levine's research revealed that using the treadmill desk burned, on average, 119 more calories per hour than sitting in an office chair. Do the math, and it's easy to see how this could potentially add up to lost weight.

Unfortunately, taking advantage of this technology currently comes at a price; retailers of treadmill desks based on Dr. Levine's vision charge anywhere from $800 to $2,500 or more for such desks. More affordable are under-the-desk pedal exercisers, which will have you pedaling away your working day. These retail for about $40.

Even then, desk-based exercisers may not be viable or practical for your work space. But if this is the case, there are many "hidden" ways to incorporate physical activity into your daily work routine, as you will see in the following pages.

So is your office culture hindering your best intentions for getting your weight under control? The signs are clear if you know what to look for. Consider the following:

◊ What is the norm in your office for birthdays? Is that "Happy Birthday" song accompanied by a cake or cookies?

◊ How about office nights out? Does your office celebrate with a pitcher of drinks every Thursday?

◊ Is there a norm for office lunches out? A favorite restaurant? And does your healthy packed lunch (if you pack one) go neglected in favor of a more tempting lunch out during these occasions?

Bear in mind that nothing is inherently "bad" about any of these activities. A song or office celebration on a birthday can go a long way in terms of making someone feel appreciated. A regularly scheduled office night out or working lunch is great for team morale. But the way these occasions are celebrated or enjoyed is often the problem.

Think, for example, about the birthday cake. A slice of birthday cake has about three hundred calories, give or take. So if you have twenty employees where you work, all of whom have birthdays, that's six thousand extra calories per year in birthday cake alone. Add in drinks, cookies, and other treats enjoyed during these gatherings, and you might discover that these "special occasions" are a huge yearly source of calories! The same applies for the weekly night out at the bar. Take into account the average number of alcoholic drinks you consume on these outings, and multiply it by fifty. Now multiply that number by the number of calories in each drink. What you find may surprise you.

The point of the examples above is not a lesson in calorie counting. Rather, they show how the pressure to be part of the team can often mean pressure to fit in and indulge. It may happen subconsciously, or if you do notice it, you may feel that you have a black-and-white choice, Do you want to be true to your healthy resolutions, or do you want to be part of the team?

Your Office Environment

The physical environment of your office, along with your work routine and your office culture, can be considered a third pillar of factors that affect your weight and health at work.

Next time you are in your office or workplace, look around. Do you and others use the stairs instead of the elevators? Do you even know where the stairs are? These considerations may seem trivial at first, but over the long run, the bouts of physical activity provided by a simple trip up or down the stairs can add up. In fact, a number of institutions have enacted initiatives to encourage the use of stairs within buildings. These initiatives are sometimes as simple as poster campaigns; others go so far as to improve the aesthetic appearance of stairwells and steps to attract more foot traffic.

Your office environment may contain other features that can more overtly affect health. Office gyms, the layout and options at the cafeteria, the location and quantity of junk-food vending machines in your building—all of these elements of the physical landscape can play a part in the decisions you make throughout the day that affect your weight.

Another important aspect of your office environment is how long you are actually at the office. For those working longer than normal hours, any negative effects the workplace may hold for weight and health will likely be magnified. But a number of studies suggest that those who work late or irregular shifts may also be at special risk of obesity and heart problems. In just one example of this link, a study in the journal *PLoS Medicine* found that in a group of late-shift workers, the odd hours were associated with an increased risk of type 2 diabetes, which is generally accompanied by overweight and obesity.[7]

Together, the "lay of the land" within your workplace and your personal work schedule can have a very real impact on your weight. Clearly you may not be able to change many of the factors at your workplace. Perhaps there is no way for you to modify your hours if you happen to work the late shift, and you may not have the authority to physically distance your desk from tempting soda machines in your vicinity.

But as we discuss ahead, you may have more power than you think to modify your office environment—or at least modify the way you interact with it. Small steps can, in the long run, add up to positive changes, and in time, you may be able to share these changes with your colleagues as well.

Taking Action at Work

We have looked at the major factors at play within your work environment and their potential influence on your weight. We have completed an assessment of your workplace that should give you an idea of what you are starting with. Now is the time to look at what you can do—and even more important, what you can influence—to make your office work for you when it comes to your weight and health.

We will begin with what you can do for yourself—the simple changes you can make unilaterally at work, involving the factors over which you have the most control. We will then expand outward to look at what you can do with regard to your office norms and office environment. Finally, we will examine the ways you may be able to influence the policies within your workplace.

You may have to start small, and that's okay; the obesogenic factors in your place of work were not built in a day, so it's not likely you as an employee can change everything drastically and immediately. Your goal, rather, should be to pave the way for modest improvements first, for yourself and possibly for your colleagues. So if your workplace gets a solid B-in healthfulness, what can you do to bring the grade up to a B+ or better?

Starting with Yourself

Individually, people can do much to increase their health at work, often with simple changes that can start immediately.

Get more steps: The benefits of recognizing where you can work a few

(continued on page 106)

Rate Your Workplace:
Is Your Job Making You Fat?

Now that we looked at some of the physical, social, and institutional factors at your workplace that could be influencing your weight, it is a good time to see how all of these factors stack up—particularly if your work environment is doing more to hurt your weight control efforts than you realized.

Below is a brief, nonscientific questionnaire. The answers you provide may help serve as a quick-and-dirty guide to how obesogenic your work environment is as well as what the primary problem area or areas may be. Bear in mind that the vast array of weight-affecting factors between the time you clock in and the time you clock out may be much more complex than what is represented here. But your answers could still be very helpful in focusing on some of the problems.

Ready? Here we go:

1. How much of your working day is spent at your desk, in your chair, or in another sedentary situation?

   a. Over 80 percent (4 points)

   b. 50–80 percent (3 points)

   c. 20–50 percent (2 points)

   d. < 20 percent (1 point)

2. How often are unhealthy snacks, such as those brought in by your colleagues, present or nearby?

   a. Nearly all the time (4 points)

   b. About three days out of the working week (2 points)

   c. Only on rare occasions—one day per week or less (1 point)

3. How close to your working area is the nearest snack or soda vending machine?

a. On the same floor or very nearby (4 points)

b. On a different floor (2 points)

c. There is no such machine, or such machines are rarely visited (0 points)

4. How would you rate the dining options at or around your office in terms of availability of healthy fare?

   a. Primarily fast food and other unhealthy fare (4 points)

   b. Some healthy choices, but unhealthy "comfort foods" are close at hand (2 points)

   c. Very healthy (1 point)

5. Does your employer's health insurance provider offer incentives or programs for healthy lifestyle indicators and behaviors?

   a. No (4 points)

   b. Perhaps, but I have not checked yet nor have these options been explained to me (2 points)

   c. Yes (0 points)

6. Does your workplace have a gym?

   a. No (4 points)

   b. No, but it does have a special arrangement with a nearby gym (special employee discounts, for example) (2 points)

   c. Yes (0 points)

Let's take a look at your score:

If you ended up with a score of 16 points or greater, your workplace could definitely use a healthy makeover. If your score fell between 8 and 16, your place of work has some good features, but it still has a ways to go. If the score you ended up with was 8 or less, congratulations! This means that the changes you make for yourself will probably be enhanced—or at least not sabotaged—by your workplace environment.

If this score is not as low as you hoped, however, you can still cut it down. We'll show you how.

more steps into your daily routine can't be overstated. One tool that may help you is a pedometer, a small device you wear on your body that tracks the number of steps you take in a day. A particularly popular model, known as Fitbit, lets you track your daily progress on your computer. These handy devices are available at a number of electronics and gadget stores or on www.fitbit.com.

Seek healthy meal options: No matter how "nutritionally hostile" your cafeteria or eating options may be, you owe it to yourself to seek out healthier options. Go for fresh vegetables and whole grains when available, and shun larger portions. Another option is to pack your lunch each day. You'll eat better and save you a considerable amount of money each week.

Learn about healthy benefits offered by your workplace: If your office has an on-site gym, or if your employer offers a discount at a nearby health club, you owe it to yourself to check it out. Many workplaces, like Massachusetts General Hospital, have programs similar to Be Fit that can go a long way toward a healthier work routine.

Changing the Office Dynamic

The culture at your workplace can be tricky to change. After all, cherished norms involving unhealthy snacks and behaviors may be sacrosanct to those who have been there for a while. But get your colleagues on board, and you will have an automatic team to help keep you on track. Here are some things you might want to try.

Start a healthy competition: We mentioned the Fitbit above. Why not start a healthy rivalry within your office based on the number of steps you and your colleagues take in a given day? A team approach to this activity can be a natural motivator.

Change the unhealthiest office habit first: Instead of Thursday morning doughnut runs, why not bring in a fruit or vegetable plate for the office instead? If you have a weekly happy hour at the bar, try suggesting a softball game as an alternative. The trick is to substitute a tradition with another activity that still brings your office together.

Turn your work buddies into workout buddies: If you have an on-site gym, try asking around to see if anyone will be your workout partner. This will give you a person to whom you are accountable; in other words, you can be each other's motivator and personal trainer!

Seeking Help from Your Employer

At a time when almost every employer is staring down the barrel of double-digit increases in health care costs, it should come as little surprise that many are taking measures to keep their employees healthy. With health programs in place, the rate of absenteeism may be reduced, and the company may also benefit from recognition by external organizations. The international Alliance for Work-Life Progress's Work-Life Innovation Excellence Award and the American Heart Association's Fit-Friendly Worksite award help boost the employer's reputation and may improve recruitment and retention of employees. Some insurers even offer benefits to the employer if employees demonstrate success in adopting healthy habits. Bring up these points with your human resources representative when you offer the following suggestions:

Push for an employee health promotion program: Such programs are often the first step to health for many in the office, and the benefits can be considerable for employees and employers alike. A seven-year study of Vanderbilt University's employee health promotion program, for example, showed a significant improvement in physical activity among participants, with the number of those reporting exercise at least one day per week increasing from 72.7 percent in 2003 to 83.4 percent in 2009.[8]

Ask about improving dining options: Do you work in a nutritionally hostile environment? Perhaps you have never thought of it this way, but if the only options are high calorie and high fat, the health threat could be real. A low-cost and effective strategy for your employer might be something like the Choose Well, Eat Well program rolled out at Massachusetts General Hospital in 2010. The program is simple: Color-coded flags denote which foods are healthy and which are not. At MGH, this measure was enough to encourage patrons to purchase more healthy and fewer unhealthy foods—and earn publication of the results in the *American Journal of Public Health*.[9]

Press for incentive programs: Does your workplace offer a program that pays employees for good health? Such programs have become more common in recent years, as the incentive for both employers and insurance companies to keep workers healthy is tremendous. If your workplace does not offer such a program, it doesn't hurt to ask.

Thinfluence Action Plan: Making Your Workplace Work for Your Weight

Your interactions and routines within the workplace are, in many ways, a perfect illustration of the concept underlying Thinfluence. Not only does the workplace environment fold in a number of social elements, it also involves your physical environment and company policies that play a powerful role in your health.

We've shown you the many ways these factors influence you; now it is your turn to apply your influence to create a healthier work environment for yourself and your colleagues.

ANALYZE

1. Which of the following best describes the physical environment of your workplace?

    A. My physical environment at work makes it difficult to be anything but sedentary; as a result I spend most of my time sitting at my desk or in my work space. There are few if any features like staircases or standing desks that encourage physical activity, and there is little opportunity to take a break for a quick walk or stretch.

B. My office or work space offers at least a few opportunities for physical activity over the course of the day. Perhaps it is relatively easy to take the stairs rather than the elevator, or outdoor areas around the workplace offer opportunities for a bit of easy exercise in the middle of the day.

C. It is clear that my office or work space is designed with activity in mind. Whether it is an on-site gym, convenient and well-lit stairwells, or other amenities, the physical environment in which I work makes it easy for me to spend time out of the office chair.

2. Which of the following best describes the social environment of your workplace?

A. My co-workers are clearly a poor influence on lifestyle-related behaviors in the workplace. They routinely bring unhealthy foods into the office to celebrate birthdays, holidays—or even for no particular reason. None of those with whom I work tend to encourage me or others to get more physical activity, and no organized activities within or outside the office foster more healthful behaviors.

B. My co-workers do not hamper the healthful efforts of those around them, but neither do they support them. The occasional cake or plate of cookies shows up in the break room on special days, but healthier fare sometimes makes an appearance as well. And while not everyone seems to enjoy regular physical activity, one or two seem to prioritize walking, sports, or some other form of exercise.

C. Many of the people I work with practice healthy activity and diet habits, and they tend to encourage the healthy efforts of others. There may even be a group exercise effort among those in my office, such as a softball team or a walking group.

3.   Which of the following best describes the policies at your place of work that affect lifestyle habits?

   A. Few if any policies encourage or reinforce healthy lifestyle choices. My employer does not offer any subsidies for gym memberships, and no incentives are provided by my employer or health insurance company to reinforce efforts to achieve good physical health.

   B. My company supports healthy lifestyles in some ways, such as offering incentives for joining a gym or sponsoring occasional events and/or seminars encouraging weight-healthy behaviors. I feel that they could be doing more, but it is a good start.

   C. In my opinion, my company's policies are a model for encouraging behaviors that lead to a better weight. Incentives are in place to reward healthy actions, and the company frequently hosts events that focus on positive lifestyle changes.

ACT

Take a look at your answers to these questions. What do you see?

◊ Mostly As: It's pretty clear that your place of work is less than ideal where your weight goals are concerned. What you can do to change the situation might be less obvious at this point. It may seem at first that you have little direct control over what happens at your office, but you can take steps to help yourself first. Take the stairs instead of the elevator and plant healthy snacks around your area to help you avoid tasty temptations that make their way through the office doors. Once you have established some healthy practices, you can start finding ways to influence others to get on board.

◊ Mostly Bs: Count yourself lucky—it seems that some good things are already happening at your office to help make it easier to achieve your weight goals. The trick now is to make the best of what you can find. That might mean asking your co-workers how to join their softball team or making sure to participate in every available program that encourages or incentivizes healthy behaviors. Your workplace may not be the healthiest place to spend the day, but you could be doing a lot worse.

◊ Mostly Cs: Workplaces as healthy as yours are rare indeed! But are you taking full advantage of what is offered? Make sure you get yourself involved in the activities of your co-workers. Know all you can about the incentive programs offered at your workplace. Even if you happen to be in the healthiest work environment, it still takes your full participation to make it work for you.

You can take a number of other actions—some small and immediate, others broader and longer term—to help improve the dynamics between where you work and what you weigh. Here are a few suggestions to get you started:

◊ Find a Thinfluencer in your workplace. This should be a person who makes the right choices involving diet, exercise, and attitude. Engage them in the process of raising the bar both for yourself and for your co-workers. Asking them to be part of a group and following their lead is a great way of acknowledging their ongoing commitment to better health.

◊ Over the next month, form a small group to try and help each other make the right choices. Together you can devise and decide on possible steps to take to get moving and eat better. Sometimes this can mean improving the environment if the workplace is cooperative, in ways such as improving the food service and places to get physical activity during breaks, or it can mean working around the existing environment, such as brown bagging, sharing lunches, and starting up walking groups.

◊ In the next few days, schedule a meeting to speak to your human resources officer about what your company offers that could help you improve your weight. Don't be shy about reminding this person that health promotion programs boost productivity, minimize absenteeism, and lead to reduced turnover of employees. Leadership can work through organizations such as the American Heart Association or a health business consultant to help retool the culture of the organization and head it in a healthier direction.

◊ If you are "lucky" enough to be in the job-hunting mode, look to see if the employer has been designated as a "fit-friendly" company. Companies receiving this distinction typically offer discounted memberships to health clubs or do this through the insurance products offered to employees, make healthy food choices available on the premises, offer education programs to employees, and even offer incentives for participation in weight loss and healthy nutrition programs.

INFLUENCE

How might the positive outcomes from the lifestyle changes you make play out at the office? Your healthy choices may have a beneficial effect on your colleagues and workplace, in turn increasing your own chances of success:

◊ Improved health and better weight control

◊ A better, healthier work environment for you and your colleagues

◊ Financial incentives for healthier behaviors

Use these positive outcomes as your motivation, as well as motivation for those with whom you work.

Finding—or Creating—Your Healthiest Workplace Possible

Looking back on her experiences with the Be Fit program, Jennifer notes that she always knew what she needed to do but felt that her work situation prevented her from getting to where she needed to be.

"I realized while talking with my dietitian that it's really funny how what you know and what you do are two totally different things," she says. "I always knew what needed to be done—stress reduction, getting my weight down, exercising more. I just couldn't do it on my own."

These days, even though the program has ended, Jennifer continues to incorporate ten to fifteen minutes of walking into her morning commute by parking a pleasant mile-long walk from the office. Her choices at work—what to eat, taking the stairs instead of the elevator—have become her routine. And she says that taken together, these small changes at work have added up to big results.

"I think the program really got me started," Jennifer says. "I know what I need to do now, and I know I can do it."

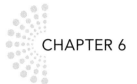

CHAPTER 6

Your Food Environment and How It Influences Your Weight

When you read the word *environment*, what comes to mind? Perhaps you think of your natural surroundings—trees, rivers, soil. Generally speaking, you are likely to think about the resources all of us need to stay alive.

This is why the term *food environment* could seem a bit confusing at first. After all, isn't the natural "environment" for your food the plate in front of you or the tip of your fork?

In fact, your food environment encompasses far more than your dining room table, your kitchen, or the inside of your home. It is the sum total of all of the food resources within your reach. With this in mind, it is easy to see how important and influential this concept can be, both for you and for those who share this environment with you. And while it may be easy to let your food environment fade into the backdrop of your day-to-day life, as with the other elements of our routines that we have highlighted in past chapters, our food environments can strongly influence our choices, our habits, and ultimately our waistlines and our health.

One example of the power of the food environment to influence weight can be seen in the story of Melarie Iron Moccasin, who was introduced to the country by Diane Sawyer in an ABC *World News* "Hidden

America" special. Thirty-year-old Melarie grew up on the Pine Ridge Indian reservation in South Dakota. The vast reservation, about the size of Delaware and Rhode Island combined, suffers from a one-two punch that, unfortunately, is not so uncommon in areas throughout the country and the world. First, it is a low-income community. Second, it lacks convenient access to healthy and affordable food as defined by the US Department of Agriculture. This combination of disadvantages has earned the reservation an unfortunate distinction as a "food desert"—a large area where there are few if any supermarkets, let alone sources of fresh fruits, vegetables, and other healthy foods. These areas are nutritionally bare wastelands dotted with a spare few widely placed oases that are often well out of the geographical or financial reach of those who live there.

In the case of the 2.2-million-acre Pine Ridge Reservation, one large supermarket exists. Because it is so remotely located, stocking this supermarket comes with added costs, thus elevating the price of many staple foods across the reservation. This, unfortunately, elevates the ingredients needed for healthy meals to luxury status—too expensive and too inconvenient for many in the financially depressed community to buy regularly.

As a result, many families on the reservation rely on whatever is available at convenience stores—a selection that is far from balanced and is often flanked by sugary sodas. This takes a toll on the health and the weight of many of the reservation's inhabitants. Melarie, ABC News found, was no exception. At her heaviest, She weighed more than 350 pounds, likely due at least in part to the difficult nutritional situation where she lived.

For years this was the reality on Pine Ridge Reservation. Then a certain well-known sandwich franchise opened its doors on the reservation. The opening of a chain sandwich restaurant would offer little, if any, change to the landscape of weight and health in nearly any other community in the United States. But in this particular food desert, this one shop, through the meals it offered, provided the reservation something that had not been available before: a convenient and afford-able source of fresh vegetables.

Melarie was one of the first employees of the new restaurant, and she was also one of the first to experience the effects of its presence.

"When I started working here, I weighed my heaviest at 356 pounds," she told ABC News. "Now I weigh 177 pounds. So altogether I lost 178 pounds."

As Melarie's weight dropped, so did her blood sugar levels. Her activity level increased, and she started to adopt healthy habits that allowed her to fight the prevailing current of obesity within her reservation.

Melarie's community is just one of many across the country and the world where the availability and cost of healthy food seem to predispose many toward an unhealthy weight. But her success reveals the power that one simple change to the food environment can have on the weight fortunes of those within an entire community.

Food deserts are not the only challenging environments that one can face. In fact, another suboptimal food environment could be described as the opposite of a food desert—what some have termed a "food swamp," but what we call a "food jungle." Those living in food jungles are surrounded by a dazzling variety of foods—mostly processed and cheap—that are almost always within reach. Divide a food jungle into its component biomes, and you are likely to find mall food courts, gas stations, drugstores, train stations, convenience stores, and super-markets, all rife with fattening and unhealthy temptations. In these environments, the worst creations of the food industry are realized, the products of the billions of dollars spent on designing foods to be maxi-mally seductive by manipulating the saltiness, sweetness, and mouth-feel. Tantalizingly packaged and conspicuously placed where you are likely to see them, these options are heavily marketed to maximize their sales. And in food jungles, they may be the only options readily visible to consumers.

But the term *food environment* does not only describe the vast geographical swaths that we think of as food deserts and food jungles. Hostile food environments can be much more local, spanning the space of a small town or several city blocks. Our own neighborhoods, for example, are food environments that can exert considerable influence over our food choices in a way that might go completely unnoticed in the course

The Economics of Your Food Environment

Your food environment is strongly influenced by various economic factors such as personal income, food affordability in your immediate area, and even the socioeconomic landscape of your community. Still, while we can say these connections exist, the nature of this relationship is quite complicated. Here are some of the widely held assumptions about money, food, and obesity— as well as some of the considerations we should bear in mind as we explore them.

Living near cheap fast food increases your risk of obesity: Fast-food restaurants, with their array of tasty, low-cost, high-calorie options in attractive packages, are a common target of blame for unhealthy food environments. Indeed, research and common sense suggest this reputation is not altogether undeserved; the presence of fast-food outlets ensures that high-calorie, high-fat options will always be available, usually with at least sixteen ounces of sugary soda thrown in. But a few studies have suggested that the location of these relatively cheap, unhealthy options in residential communities is only modestly associated with a community's obesity rates[1,2,3]— which means that this is not the only factor at play.

Having a full-scale supermarket nearby ensures a healthy diet: The good news is that large supermarkets often offer healthy foods at reasonable prices. The bad news? A large proportion of the products that are on special or for which you have clipped a coupon are junk food. Sound surprising? Take a look next time you are browsing the of your daily routine, because some sources of the food that makes up your diet are just a bit more convenient, albeit quite a bit more fattening. Even the food environment we create within our homes—inside our own pantries and cabinets, on the coffee table that sits between the sofa and the television—can be a powerful factor in the decisions we make

aisles. Since large grocery stores also increase availability of unhealthy foods, simply having these stores nearby is no assurance that you will be eating any healthier.

Eating healthy is expensive if you live in most communities: If you happen to be among the relative few who live on a farm or near one, the chances are higher that you will have a relatively easy time finding fresh, healthy food at a reasonable price. This may not be the case if you live in a suburban or urban environment where a premium is often placed on fresh, unprocessed options—particularly in stores that specialize in organic food and at farmers' markets. That's not to say that strategies to eat healthy on a smaller budget are impossible to come by; however, if you live in these areas, eating healthy on a budget will probably be a challenge.

Conversely, eating unhealthy is usually cheap: Convenient, quick, and cheap is a common mantra for some of the more unhealthy options available to us in our day-to-day environments. If the food environment at your workplace, for example, is dotted with vending machines, chances are high that you will see them as a quick and easy way to get rid of your hunger for about a dollar. Living in a neighborhood with a convenience store means that your morning regimen may include a daily coffee and doughnut for a buck or two. In the big picture, however, it may be surprising to see how expensive these unhealthy routines can actually be— not just in the immediate sense, but in the form of obesity and long-term health effects. A study by Walter and his colleagues published in the *American Journal of Clinical Nutrition* supports this point as well as the previous one.[4] On average, it is true that the healthfulness of a person's diet correlates with cost. But at any cost, Walter and his colleagues found, some people eat a healthy diet and others eat a diet that is far from healthy. So it may not be all about the money after all.

unconsciously every day about food. And we may not recognize the impact of these decisions until the next time we step onto the scale. If we ever recognize it at all.

In this chapter, we will be shining a light on all components of the food environment. More important, we will show you the ways that you can use your influence to improve your food environment, whether it is inside your home, in your immediate neighborhood, or in your community as a whole. Regardless of where you are starting in terms of your overall food environment, these simple steps will help you set the stage for a healthier weight.

Do It Today: Four Simple Food Environment "Home Improvements"

The steps you take toward a healthier home food environment need not be extreme. Here are four small steps you can take today.

Ditch the sugary soda: It may seem simple, but for some households this may be easier said than done. A Gallup poll, the results of which were published in July 2012, found that nearly half of Americans drink soda daily. This despite the fact that most of us certainly know by now that drinking it regularly is not the best thing we could be doing for ourselves. While plain water is an ideal alternative, many other low-calorie or no-calorie alternatives exist that might soften the blow of a no-cola policy in your home. Club soda, for instance, gives the same fizzy feeling with no calories. Add a bit of lemon or lime, and you may not have the sugary jolt you had before, but you will still have a refreshing beverage in your hand.

Banish bad foods to the back: Is it all too easy to reach for sugary snacks when you want them? Consider relocating these snacks to a less-convenient area of the fridge, cabinets, or kitchen pantry. In their

Your Home Food Environment

We opened this chapter by discussing a food environment in the broadest sense—one that reaches over an entire extended community. But the first environment where you will likely exert your influence may be a place you do not often think of as a food environment per se. This environment is your kitchen, your living room, and the other areas of your home where you eat your meals and snacks.

In many ways, the concept of your food environment parallels the Circles of Influence model (page 10). While the influences from your

place, substitute healthier options—fresh-cut vegetables and fruit, refreshing yogurt, or whole wheat snacks. Knowing that the less-healthy snacks are still available may help make the switch seem less restrictive, but you will also know that a healthy option is always close at hand. On the other hand, some of us find it easier to just keep the cookies and candy out of the house because our ability to resist temptation is too low.

Out with the white foods, in with the brown: One of the easiest swaps you can make in your cupboard may be whole grain pasta and brown rice instead of their refined counterparts. These sources of carbohydrates are more filling and

more nutritious, and they provide more nutrients with your meals. It may be an adjustment at first, but you might find that the change is worth making.

Capitalize on your free time to set yourself up to succeed: When you *aren't* hungry and have your food "wits" about you, prepare fruits, veggies, and protein snacks so that you can simply pick them up and go in the morning. Brown rice can be prepared, boiled, and frozen in individual containers and then warmed up during the week to accompany a healthy protein choice and some greens. Taking this extra time in advance helps minimize your excuses for not choosing wisely when it comes to nutrition.

immediate neighborhood—as well as those from the larger community to which it belongs—will undoubtedly play a role in your daily choices, the choices you make in your environment at home have the greatest impact on your weight and the weight of those with whom you live. Likewise, you will probably find that making changes in your home food environment is an accessible goal, and it will have more immediate results than any changes you attempt in the broader food environment—at least to begin with.

How can you tell if you have a positive or negative food environment at home? The proof is in the pudding . . . that is, if that pudding happens to be stacked by the case in your pantry or refrigerator. These are a couple of the places in your home that determine the likelihood that your home environment will lead to weight gain and obesity. Other areas include those within arm's length of where you spend time relaxing—whether it is in front of the TV, in your bedroom, or elsewhere. What do you see when you look in these areas? Is there an abundance of fresh vegetables and healthy whole grains for meal preparation, and veggies and fruits for snacking? Or do you find bags of potato chips, sugary sodas, and products rich in sugar and refined starch?

Not all signs of an unhealthy food environment at home are quite as obvious as a brightly colored cellophane bag of fattening snacks, of course. Many foods in your pantry traditionally associated with preparing healthy, hearty meals are also linked to higher rates of weight gain than are other foods. This point is demonstrated in a study in the *New England Journal of Medicine* to which Walter contributed.[5]

Consider, for example, the humble potato. As it turns out, regular consumption of potatoes, more than any other food, had a stronger link to weight gain over time. In fact, Walter and his colleagues found that regular potato consumption packs on an average of 1.3 pounds over a four-year period—and that's not counting eating them in their popular chip form. Red meat and processed meats, too, were linked to weight gain over time, but they still trailed the potato in terms of obesogenic potential.

Does this mean that to lose weight, we need to make our homes a completely potato-free zone? Spud lovers, whose knuckles might go white at this thought, can ease their grip on this book since this is almost never the case. But it does tell us that it makes sense to reexamine the options we have in our home food environment. The same study found that adding daily servings of other foods—fruit and nuts, for example, or vegetables—was actually associated with a bit of weight *loss* each year.

So it's not hard to imagine what might happen if you swapped out a few of those potatoes in your pantry for fruits and nuts instead. We are proposing small changes to your food environment, modest adjustments to what is easily accessible in your home. Make these tweaks, and you may find that you put your family's healthy choices on autopilot: You have created a food environment in which healthier eating and snacking have become the norm. More important, however, you will be influencing your family to look for healthier options in the food environment outside of the home as well. As long as you try to do the right things and set the best examples in your home, you and your loved ones will tend to gravitate toward more healthy choices, no matter the community in which you happen to live.

Avoiding a "Hostile" Food Environment at Home

One important caveat to bear in mind while you are set on improving your home food environment is to make sure that, in your zeal to help your family eat healthier, you do not introduce an overly restrictive food environment. Control that environment too tightly, and your family members—and even you—may end up searching outside of your home for the unhealthy foods you crave.

Try starting small and make changes gradually. Before long, healthier choices may gradually take over your routine, bit by bit.

The Food Environment in Your Neighborhood

It's time to step outside your front door to look at the food environment in your immediate neighborhood. What food sources are around the corner or down the street? Of those that are in your neighborhood, which ones do you frequent? Or are there any sources of food in your neighborhood?

If you live in an urban setting, it is possible that you are a relatively short walk or bus ride away from several restaurants, a grocery store or two, and a few corner bodegas. A suburbanite may be a mile or so away from the nearest dining options or grocery stores, but significantly closer to a convenience store. If you live in a rural environment, however, it is possible that you need to jump into your car and drive many miles to find a source of food that is not your own pantry or cellar.

As you can see, a wide variety of neighborhood food environments exist, and all of us learn fairly quickly how best to adapt these environments to our budgets, lifestyle preferences, and schedules.

But the choices we make are not always the healthiest. As it turns out, convenience is a key factor for most of us—and prioritizing convenience first, it turns out, may be worse for our waistlines than we believe at first blush.

Let's look at the example of the urban neighborhood. In a recent study published in the *American Journal of Public Health*, Diane Gibson, PhD, of The City University of New York, demonstrated that in city environments, those who lived close to smaller grocery stores—which are thought to have many unhealthy food options—tended to be heavier than those who did not.[6]

While this research only shows an association (not necessarily that proximity to unhealthy food choices causes weight gain), it does underscore an interesting yet understandable idea: that the more convenient an option is to us, the more likely we will be to choose it. Given our busy modern schedules, it should come as little surprise that we are more likely to choose the path of least resistance on most days when it comes to food—unless, of course, we are consciously making the decision to do something healthy for ourselves.

What this means for someone living in a suburban environment is that, at the end of a long day at work, a quick trip to the neighborhood drive-thru may appear much more appealing to us than stopping at a supermarket on the way home to buy healthy ingredients and then going home to put effort into preparing a healthy, nutritious, weight-friendly meal.

If this sounds like a familiar routine to you, don't feel too bad about it. This decision is often made on a purely subconscious level, and in most cases it is made in the interest of time. But the fact remains that the convenience of our surroundings is a powerful influence, and it can be a formidable saboteur in our efforts to make a healthy change. It is particularly important to realize how convenience can be an important ingredient in habits. Bow to convenience often enough, and you will eventually find that what was once an occasional indulgence has become a routine—as bad luck would have it, the kind of routine that has the potential to show up on your waistline before too long.

So is it possible for us to influence our way out of this potentially obesogenic convenience trap set by our neighborhood food environment—and if so, how? Part of the solution may be discussing with your family, neighbors, and friends who live nearby the particular challenges that your neighborhood poses. What solutions have worked for them? What pitfalls have they identified? Knowing what they know and sharing what you have learned could help all of you approach your neighborhood food environment more intelligently.

A very concrete solution that could arise from these discussions, particularly if you are close with your neighbors, is a neighborhood vegetable garden. In addition to fostering closer neighborhood ties, a common project like a garden is a way to ensure that you have a steady supply of fresh, seasonal vegetables for many months out of the year, with a minimal impact on your pocketbook. This solution takes a bit of time and organization, but once it gets rolling, you may find that the support and motivation you get from others who are involved is enough to keep the good food coming.

If you and your neighbors lack green thumbs, you can interact more widely with your greater food environment and still ensure a steady supply of fresh, seasonal produce. Community Supported Agriculture programs, or CSAs for short, allow you to buy a recurring "share" of food from a regional farmer. For a modest up-front payment, you and your neighbors can split a share or several shares—often regardless of whether you live in a less-than-ideal food environment or not. (To learn more about CSAs in your area, visit www.localharvest.org/csa/.)

Could your influence in improving the neighborhood food environment lead to a better weight for you as well as your neighbors? Better yet, could these same actions create a self-sustaining community project that could keep you and your family engaged and eating more healthily? It's a perfect embodiment of the Thinfluence concept, and with the right approach and support within your neighborhood, it may very well succeed.

Your Community Food Environment: Oasis, Desert, or Jungle?

Returning to Melarie's story, the Pine Ridge Reservation example at the beginning of this chapter is powerful because it shows what can happen when the entire region where you live presents a challenging food environment. Research has shown that millions like Melarie live in this country—entire communities—and face these challenges. In 2011, Debra Reed, PhD, and other researchers at Texas Tech University looked at the rural side of the problem in a report in the *Journal of Nutrition Education and Behavior*. Their findings suggested that specific conditions brought about by geographical location conspire with diet and poor physical activity, exposing entire communities to risk factors for weight gain.[7] What's more, several researchers have found that food deserts are not confined to rural areas—a fact demonstrated by Cynthia Gordon, PhD, and colleagues with the New York City Department of Public Health when they documented the factors contributing to urban food deserts in East Harlem and North Brooklyn.[8]

If you happen to live in a food desert or a food jungle, what are your options? The key in this case, it turns out, is to take advantage of whatever influence you can gather within your neighborhood to encourage positive changes within your community.

Say, for example, that you have used your healthy influence to help your neighbors to adopt various weight-friendly behaviors—a community garden or a neighborhood rotation for healthy food trips. This could be your chance to see the Thinfluence concept at work. Small groups of people, working toward the common goal of a healthier life, have the potential to make a big impact on community policies and practices. If the stores in your area are food jungles with little or no healthy fare, you and others from your neighborhood may want to approach these stores and ask them to carry specific, healthier products. (This, by the way, is a strategy that Walter has used several times to get stores close to where he lives to stock Kashi whole grain pilaf.) The tactic works best if multiple people ask, so communicating with your friends and neighbors about it can help.

With a little help from those in your neighborhood, you may even succeed in working through local government to get grocery stores located in places where they are absent. Walter's community used this approach—and successfully at that—after a major supermarket near the neighborhood shut down and the community found itself in the middle of a food desert. With neighborhood encouragement, the city government made significant efforts to get other grocery stores to fill the gap. Today there are three options where there were once none.

Properly organized neighborhood efforts can also be used to limit fast-food outlets near schools and can even offer support to many of the efforts now under way in some cities. Many of these efforts come in the form of programs like CSAs and community-supported farmers' markets. Other initiatives take aim at known contributors to obesity. Because of the strong evidence that high soda consumption is contributing to the epidemics of obesity and diabetes, Boston has now banned the sale of soda on all city property. New York City has passed regulations limiting the size of sugary beverages that can be sold at restaurants and movie theaters. Your small neighborhood could wield substantial influence on such efforts—and these efforts, in turn, could make your community, neighborhood, and home places where it is easier to maintain a healthy weight.

Weight and the School Environment

If you are a parent, understanding the food environment at your child's school is important. In many ways, the similarities between the school food environment and the community food environment are obvious: a regular daily schedule with predetermined dining options.

Likewise, there may be opportunities for you to influence the system to improve the health of the school environment both for your child and for other children. Clearly you will not be able to follow your child to class and encourage their buddies to eat carrots instead of Ho Hos (and pity be upon your child if you are the type of parent to try). But by engaging with administrators and others in power, you may be able to influence them to look at the following areas:

Healthy cafeteria options: The issue of unhealthy school lunches was brought to the fore by Jamie Oliver, whose *Food Revolution* TV show revealed to millions the various institutional, economic, and political influences that determine what your child puts in his or her mouth. It's unlikely that you have the time or resources to launch a similar effort, but that does not mean you can't ask those in charge of your schools to consider healthier options for the children they serve.

Out with vending machines and in with fresh water bubblers: Does your child's school have vending machines accessible to students? These can be a tempting source of empty calories for kids.

Thinfluence Action Plan:
Your Food Environment

Few of us are fortunate enough to live in an environment that completely supports healthy weight maintenance or weight loss. So if you live in a food

Ask administrators what school policies are with regard to student access. Ideally, schools would not have vending machines (many of us managed to get an education without them), but one alternative is to push for the unhealthy options in vending machines to be replaced with healthier snacks. HUMAN Healthy Vending is a nonprofit company that seeks to promote such swaps; learn more about them at www.healthyvending.com/aboutus/.

Unfortunately many schools do not have easy access to the best option: a drinking fountain with free tap water. Making sure these are a conspicuous part of the school environment should be a top parental priority. It is worth noting that across the country, parents' groups have traditionally succeeded in getting rid of soda in schools. These efforts, started locally, eventually went statewide. Now they exist as a national agreement coordinated by the Clinton Foundation. Parent power!

Push for PE: This point touches on another concept: the physical environment. While we will be dealing with this more in depth in the chapters to come, it is important to recognize the interplay between physical environment and the food environment, particularly where the school setting is concerned. Physical education classes are an endangered species in school curricula across the country. This is unfortunate, because much is to be said for their importance. Not only does physical activity make for healthier kids, but one review of studies published in the *Archives of Pediatrics and Adolescent Medicine* showed that kids engaging in physical activity tended to perform better academically as well.[9] Learn about the opportunities for physical activity at your child's school and see if they can be improved.

desert or a food jungle, take comfort in the fact that you are not alone.

But given what we have discussed in this chapter, it is clear that you have the power to take meaningful action to change the food environment—whether it is in your own home, within your immediate neighborhood, or in your town or city. Once you have opened your eyes to the food environment in which you live, you can start using your influence to take action.

ANALYZE

1. How would you describe your home food environment?

   A. The layout of my home seems to encourage unhealthy choices. Whenever I open the fridge or a cupboard door in my kitchen, junk food is likely to be the first thing that I see. Candy bowls, cookie jars, and other sources of temptation are fixtures in other rooms as well—particularly in the places where I spend most of my leisure time. Whole and fresh ingredients are in short supply, and most of the meals I would prepare myself are of the packaged, heat-and-eat variety. Healthy foods? Not in this house.

   B. A pretty even mix of healthy and unhealthy food choices are within easy reach in my home. I usually manage to keep my kitchen stocked with at least some fresh fruits and vegetables, as well as other healthy snacks. However, snack cakes and chips are still regular fixtures in the pantry, and a bottle of soda or two are always in the fridge.

   C. Fresh, whole foods are the norm in my home. Sugary, processed foods are rarely seen, and if they are present they are usually banished to the back of the cabinets so they are not the first option I come across when in a snacking mood. Areas of the home not designated for eating purposes are kept free of unhealthy foods, for the most part.

2. How would you describe the food environment in your immediate neighborhood?

A. Few if any places within a ten-minute walk, bicycle ride, or drive from my home would be considered a source of healthy, affordable food.

B. My neighborhood has at least one or two places where I can find nutritious food, such as a grocery store. They may not be the most convenient options around, but with a little effort I can get what I need.

C. My neighborhood is a veritable cornucopia of healthy food options! In addition to one or two well-stocked grocery stores, I am close to a farmers' market, a community garden, or some other source of fresh produce.

3. What about your community at large? How would you describe the greater food environment in the city, town, or county in which you live?

A. Aside from convenience stores and a few restaurants, my community has few fresh, healthy food options. Stocking up usually takes some effort—such as driving to the next community, for example, or taking a bus for more than thirty minutes.

B. My community has a fair assortment of grocery stores, and I can usually find what I need to prepare decent meals at home. However, good produce and other fresh foods are sometimes hard to come by, and finding them in town is only an occasional treat.

C. My community not only has an assortment of places that offer staples but is also home to a vast spectrum of options. From fresh fish and lean meats to produce and grains, I am spoiled with choices.

ACT

Take a moment to consider your answers to the questions. What do your answers look like?

◊ **Mostly As:** In your overall food environment, it is clear that you face challenges that many others do not. If the problem is within your neighborhood or community—for example, if you live in a food desert—the challenge that lies before you is to create an oasis in your own home. How can you increase the healthfulness of your home food environment? One option might be to get together with those who live near you to form a neighborhood group that can pool together on grocery trips. Setting up a grocery rotation like this, in which everyone takes turns picking up food for everyone else, may turn out to be an efficient approach for everyone involved—and since everyone ends up saving money on gas, it is affordable as well. Also, if you have limited access to a grocery store, buying more frozen vegetables may make sense. These healthy options are not perishable, and they can be relatively inexpensive if bought in bulk. If the problem is in your home food environment, the solution may be even simpler—it's time to reorganize your pantry to make healthy options more readily accessible than unhealthy foods. This may mean loading the areas you visit most with healthier foods such as fruits, vegetables, nuts, and whole grain cereals. You can start this strategy as soon as your next visit to the grocery store. Stock your home with healthier foods, cut out the junk, and give yourself three weeks to complete your kitchen overhaul.

◊ **Mostly Bs:** Most people are at this starting point, so you are in good company. The challenge for you will be to make the extra effort to improve your food environment, even if you feel that it is "good enough for now." Do a bit of homework to better understand the options in your neighborhood or community. You may be surprised to find a farmers' market that you never knew about or another source of fresh foods. You may even want to start your own garden! The more small improvements you can make, the less likely that you will turn to fattening or highly processed foods. Give it a bit of thought—your bathroom scale will thank you.

◊ **Mostly Cs:** Lucky, lucky . . . you appear to live in a healthy food paradise! The simple trick for you is to make sure you take full advantage of what your neighborhood and community have to offer.

While your food environment at home may be good for now, it takes vigilance to keep it that way, so don't stop poking around for hidden healthy food options where you live.

Of course, no matter what your food environment happens to be, it is what you do with it that counts. Here are a couple of tips that should help anyone make the most of their existing food environment:

◊ Commit to preparing at least three dinners a week, focusing on healthy ingredients and reasonable portions. Recipes are a must; set a goal to find three healthy recipes per week. Better yet, enlist your family and friends to help.

◊ Even if time is tight, you can still make the best of your available food environment. Consider picking up a book that Walter coauthored with cookbook author Mollie Katzen, titled *Eat, Drink, and Weigh Less*. In it, you will find a plan for people who have limited time for food preparation or limited cooking facilities.

INFLUENCE

The thing to remember about food environments is that they rarely affect just you. This means that as you work to change your food environment, the benefits you reap will be visible and enjoyed by those around you. This alone may be enough to help influence others to reinforce your efforts, as an improved environment may also mean the following for all involved:

◊ Improved diet habits, a lower caloric intake, and a more ideal weight

◊ Cost savings from carpooling and buying in bulk

◊ Improved relationships and a sense of a common goal among others in your community

Remember that each of the changes you try may or may not be a useful part of your toolbox. Don't be afraid to experiment; even small changes to your food environment can help you achieve a healthier weight.

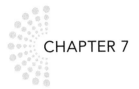

CHAPTER 7

How Your Physical Environment and Surroundings Affect Your Weight

"If it weren't for the fact that the TV set and the refrigerator are so far apart, some of us wouldn't get any exercise at all."

—JOEY ADAMS, COMEDIAN AND *NEW YORK POST* COLUMNIST

If you find yourself smiling after reading this oft-cited quote, it just might be because it rings somewhat true for you. Don't feel bad! All of us can relate to this sentiment on some level, primarily because it is so natural for our surroundings to shape our behaviors if we let them. The layout of our homes, the walkability of our neighborhoods, and the arrangement of our work spaces are powerful determinants of our activity levels and food choices. And as businessman Jack Rennes will tell you, this is even truer when the physical environment is in a constant state of flux.

On any given day, it is difficult to know what form forty-two-year-old Jack's physical environment will take—a hotel room, a rental car, a lonely airport terminal, or a business-class seat forty thousand feet in the air.

Jack runs a successful propane business in New England, and his 160 employees count on him to make the trips and connections that keep the company going. Jack, in turn, counts on fitting in time between his travels to be an involved father to his four kids. Not surprisingly, his busy schedule and his constantly changing surroundings make a regular exercise routine—or even avoiding a sedentary, obesogenic lifestyle—a challenge.

When we finally caught up with Jack, he was in the middle of business as usual: racing between appointments in a rental car, with fifteen minutes left before his next meeting, which would take place in a family-style chain restaurant.

Like so many Americans who work on the road or on unusual schedules, Jack faces the specter of a constantly shifting physical environment. Depending on where he happens to be, he has learned to expect unhealthy meals on the road, long hours in transit, and the temptations of hotel room snack bars. The fact that he is often unfamiliar with his surroundings also means no regular daily running route or set weekly routine at the neighborhood gym. Making matters worse, Jack also contends with a family history of weight problems.

"There may be other people who naturally have an incredible body. . . . I'm not that guy," he says. "Neither are any of the people who are in my family. Weight has been an issue in my family as far as I can remember, going back to when I went to Weight Watchers meetings with my parents and grandparents."

Most faced with Jack's situation would likely slip into unhealthy lifestyle patterns. And Jack readily admitted he had been there. Earlier in his professional career, he had packed on the pounds, largely due to his working lifestyle. The irony was that the more he had to travel from place to place, the less he actually moved around. From his high school wrestling weight of 168, Jack gradually saw the number on the scale rise until he hit 250 pounds. It was only then that he figured out how to incorporate physical activity into his constantly changing surroundings.

"Traveling is exceedingly tough," he says. "You have to look outside of the box. Most hotels you stop at have something there—a gym, a pool. I think you just normalize it. You can say that everything is different, but every gym environment is the same, every Y is the same, every pool is the same."

The realization that every physical environment he encountered—no matter how far away from home—had opportunities for exercise marked the turning point for Jack. Even away from the sanctuary of the hotel, Jack says he has adapted a mind-set that lets him find some way, any way, to get physical activity out of his surroundings.

In short, the world is now Jack's gym.

"At O'Hare International Airport, there are those tunnels with those stairs at the end," he says. "If I have the time between flights, that's definitely a place to walk. If there's stairs, I don't take the escalator. I will even walk laps when I'm on the phone with people, just to get my heart rate up. If you normalize that, it becomes what you do—you go and you find the place, and you just do it. You have to have that willpower, almost that habit, to do it."

Bending Your Physical Environment to Your Will

Fortunately, not all of us have jobs that, like Jack's, force us to contend with changes in our location and surroundings from one day to the next. But it is very likely that you face your own set of challenges from your physical surroundings. For any of us, each day presents thousands of different ways that our routines—and the way they affect our physical environment—can have a big effect on our ability to achieve our weight goals.

So what are we really talking about when we say "physical environment"? Defined broadly, your physical environment refers to the characteristics of your surroundings that have the potential to affect your decisions on calorie intake (in other words, eating) and calorie expenditure (in other words, activity).

In some ways, your physical environment goes hand in hand with the food environment concept that we addressed in the last chapter. Your surroundings, after all, are the backdrop for the food choices available in your home, your neighborhood, and your greater community. But the impact of your physical environment actually extends even further than this. It determines not only what you eat, but also how you eat. Additionally, your physical environment sets the parameters for how much activity you get each day, a crucial factor in your weight. And features of your physical environment shape the behaviors that affect your waistline in other, less obvious ways.

Because our physical environment has such a profound effect on the behaviors tied to our weight, the more you understand your surroundings and adapt to them, the more you will be able to tip the scales in your favor to get to your best weight. Just as in the last chapter, when we discussed numerous ways our food environment could be tweaked or modified to the benefit of our waistlines, we can change the way we interact with our surroundings to achieve the same end. And much like your food environment, you can exert your influence on your physical environment on many different levels—from the decisions you make in arranging your immediate home environment and workplace to the way you function within the other various landscapes you encounter daily.

The good news is that your approach to your physical environment can be as individual as your situation. So perhaps you are someone for whom a routine as a stay-at-home parent pretty much limits your physical environment to the areas in and around your home on most days. Or maybe you work long hours in an office, making your company's building your primary physical environment. You might be someone for whom improving the way that you interact with your physical environment means examining your daily commute to look for opportunities for more walking and less time sitting behind a wheel. Or the best strategy for you might be making the most of the resources at your neighborhood gym. Whichever situation applies to you, modifying your physical environment is probably not rocket science. The trick is to keep your eyes open for the factors in your physical environment that have an impact on your weight. After that, you simply need to put some time and thought into finding the various opportunities your physical environment presents and choose from the huge array of options you are likely to find. And that, dear readers, is where we come in.

In this chapter, we will explore the factors in your home, neighborhood, and community that may be influencing your success at achieving your desired weight. Whether they are the features in our kitchens and living rooms, the environments in which we work, or the layout of our neighborhoods and communities as a whole, these obesogenic factors can have a powerful effect—not just on your ability to achieve your weight goals, but also on the healthier weight aspirations of your family and close friends. The following pages should help you see the full picture of the various factors of your living environment that either encourage or discourage regular physical activity and healthy eating habits.

This, of course, is the big picture. As we have before, we will start in the area over which you will likely have the most direct control: your home physical environment.

Your Physical Environment at Home

Your interaction with your physical environment starts each day the moment you roll over to turn off the alarm clock (or, if you are like us, hit the snooze button a few times!) before getting out of bed. You take a set number of steps when you head into your kitchen to make breakfast, a few more steps to the bathroom, and then more still as you head out the door to your driveway or to the sidewalk outside your home. Fast-forward to the end of the day, and you take a certain number of steps from your front door to your sofa, then perhaps to your kitchen or dining area. You sit, you eat. Again to the bathroom, and again into bed to call it a night.

Humans are hardwired to develop routines for the situations we face again and again, and our physical environments set the stage for these routines. If the basic routine described above reflects your daily pattern, you are probably not thinking about how many calories you expend as you walk around inside your home or head out to the car to leave for work. And yet this is *actual* physical activity that burns *actual* calories. Now, if your morning and evening routines mirror this example, you're obviously not getting much physical activity or burning any great number of calories within your home environment. In other words, you are missing out on some opportunities.

The good news is that the way you perform the daily dance of your routine is not hardwired. It is not written in stone. Changing your physical environment at home, and how you interact with it, is well within your power.

You need to put on a new hat—that of a "home inspector." Except that instead of searching the corners of your home for the odd leak or wiring mishap, you will be sniffing out the physical features of your home that could be short-circuiting your efforts at a healthier weight.

Start with the dining space in your home. What is it used for? Is it reserved solely for Thanksgiving and other holidays? Or, more commonly, has your dining room table become a holding area for outgoing mail, magazines, catalogs, children's toys, and other various items? If either of these scenarios is the case, you and your family are probably consuming meals in areas that would be considered less than perfect for healthy eating habits— on the sofa in front of the television, for example, or straight out of an open takeout box on the kitchen counter.

It is hard to overstate the importance of your dining space in your home physical environment. The place where we eat our meals—ideally, where we *enjoy* our meals—should be comfortable, conducive to conversation, and engaging so your family will be encouraged to sit down and eat.

This was the need Malissa faced roughly three years ago when, in her words, the dining room table had become a "repository for crap" in her house. The move to change this part of her physical environment was decisive.

She cleaned off the dining room table and made a new rule: The table was to be for meals only. She removed all clutter from the rest of the room and ensured that the table was well lit and inviting. From here on out, the new household norm was to live in a home with a clean, accessible dining room table and to have nice sit-down dinners.

Dramatic changes came from this decision. The conversations and bonding that her family enjoyed over shared meals increased, and her family managed to recapture an aspect of mealtime that modern society has largely lost to changes in schedules and technology. She created a space in the home that would potentially enhance both the health of and relationships within the family—all this from the very small investment in time that it took to improve this aspect of her home physical environment.

Returning to your new role as home inspector—you may find that your own home physical environment could benefit from designating the dining area as a place that is actually 100 percent devoted to the act of dining. Teach your partner or kids that this is a special place in the home, and you will have influenced their behavior and approach to meals and eating.

As you continue your inspection, look at the way you have organized the food in your cupboards, refrigerator, and pantry. Do you have your food arranged in a way that healthier options are more easily available? The usual food storage areas of your kitchen may make it a challenge to access the healthy options first. If this is the case, reshuffle your food, changing the arrangement so the most easily accessible areas of your pantry are designated for whole grain foods. Upper shelves and harder-to-reach areas will be the new home for less-healthy foods and occasional treats. This simple change may not seem like a big deal at first glance, but the changes to your daily routine going forward thanks to these adjustments to your physical environment are likely to be noticeable.

In fact, there may be many opportunities to make these little tweaks to the physical environment around your home. And these changes are not restricted to your eating habits. A home reorganization can also lead to more physical activity. This may mean replacing your leaf blower with an old-fashioned rake to get a bit of extra exercise, or leaving your home from the front door instead of the side door each day to give yourself a few dozen extra steps to your car. The key is to increase your awareness of these potential positive changes to your routine—and make them happen.

The TV Tray: The Second-Worst Piece of Furniture You Can Own?

If you happen to come across a TV tray in the course of your "home inspection," you might do well to set it by the curb the next chance you get. It is a well-known fact among researchers in the field that when people eat while watching television, they tend not to realize how many calories they are actually consuming—an invitation for overeating. As proof of this principle, researchers at the University of Birmingham reported that those who eat in front of the television are likely to consume more calories throughout the day than those who pay more attention to what they are eating.[1]

One of the pioneers in this field is Brian Wansink, PhD, of Cornell University. Dr. Wansink, author of *Mindless Eating: Why We Eat More Than We Think*, has demonstrated in a number of experiments the eating behaviors people exhibit when they are not paying attention to what they are doing when they eat.[2,3,4] Your physical environment can play a big role in this distraction—particularly when a TV is involved. So during mealtime, it will serve you to stay away from it as much as possible.

. . . And the Worst Piece of Furniture in Your Home for Your Weight?

By far, the worst piece of "furniture" for your weight is your TV set. Sure, you may not consider this to be a piece of furniture at all. But considering the impact it could be having on your daily

The Physical Environment
of Your Community

Metropolitan areas like New York City, San Francisco, and Boston have something in common—and it's not just championship-level professional baseball teams.[6] All of them rank notably high in terms of walkability on

routine, we decided it was better not to split hairs.

Chances are, you have at least one TV somewhere in your home. And if your home is like most in the United States, you probably have more than one—you might even have a TV in each room. In the next chapter, we will discuss the messages that come out of it and how they affect your weight. But for now, let's focus purely on its impact on your physical environment.

If you want to get a better idea of how much your TVs could be affecting your daily routine, spend a week logging how much time you and your family spend seated in front of one. You may be surprised! According to the A.C. Nielsen Company, which keeps an eye on these things, the average American watches nearly five hours of TV each day. We engage in this activity religiously—and usually we are sitting down while we do it.

If you spend excessive time in front of the tube, you might very well decide to take action—perhaps by limiting television watching to only one room of your home, or by designating certain "TV-free" hours in your household. Or you may take a cue from a study out of the University of Tennessee,[5] which suggests a simple change in TV-watching routine: At every commercial break, get off the couch and start walking in place. When the commercial break stops, you can sit down again and watch your show. Simple, right? But the researchers in this study found that sticking to this simple rule during an hour and a half of TV watching burns 165 calories—essentially the equivalent of thirty minutes of walking.

Whatever you decide to do, it is worth your time to recognize the impact of your TV in your home physical environment and to find a healthier way to position it or watch it.

the popular site Walk Score (www.walkscore.com/rankings/). These three cities ranked the best out of fifty studied, in fact, in terms of proximity of residential addresses to amenities such as grocery stores, banks, parks, and entertainment.

On the opposite end of the spectrum are Oklahoma City; Charlotte, North Carolina; and Jacksonville, Florida—the metropolitan areas designated as least walkable, according to the Walk Score algorithm.

The formula Walk Score uses is not perfect, a point openly acknowledged by its designers. For example, the score does not take into account traffic threats to pedestrians or the size and quality of sidewalks. But what it does very well is underscore a very important aspect of a neighborhood's physical environment: how the degree of physical activity we get within our immediate neighborhood surroundings depends almost entirely on how conveniently we can walk from place to place to get what we need. If you are fortunate enough to live in a home that is close to the amenities you desire, you will naturally walk there and back more often than you drive, and you will burn more calories in your daily or weekly routine as an added benefit. If, however, you live in a city scoring low on the Walk Score scale—or, more likely, if you live in a suburban or rural area where the nearest amenities are miles away—the chances that regular walking will be part of your daily chores are fairly slim.

The effect of walkable neighborhoods on our weight is not just an academic idea—it bears out in real life. This is what researchers at the University of Utah found when they compared the addresses of more than 450,000 people living in and around Salt Lake City with their body mass index scores.[7] As the walkability of a neighborhood within this metro area increased, the risk of being overweight decreased for the people living in that neighborhood. The researchers also found that the more people in a neighborhood walked to work instead of driving a car, the lower the risk was of obesity for any particular individual in that neighborhood.

The problem many of us face, of course, is that we do not live in a neighborhood or environment where walking to work, to the grocery store, or to various other amenities is an option. Even for those who live in urban environments, where walkable areas tend to be more common, the expansion of many metropolitan areas across the country has led to the rise of sprawling suburbs and bedroom communities—and along with them, distances between homes and amenities that make an automobile a necessity. The relationship between our physical environment and our transportation choices is important. It is easy to see how a thirty-minute walk or bike ride to work is a natural opportunity for extra exercise, whereas a thirty-minute-each-way commute in your driver's seat will add an hour per day to your sedentary time.

Lack of walkability is not the only factor with potential to make your neighborhood physical environment less compatible with a healthy weight. Security of the areas around your home and work is also an element of the physical environment. So, too, are factors such as noise and air pollution. If you are in an area where the climate is not conducive to outdoor activities for months on end, that too can be a barrier to activity and is thus a factor to consider within the physical environment.

Not all of these factors are easily changed. No matter what kind of influence you wield, for example, you can't control the weather where you live. For this reason, however, it is important for us to find the features of our neighborhood physical environment that are conducive to weight-healthy behaviors and overcome these barriers.

For example, even if your neighborhood makes it impossible for you to walk or bike to work, you may still be able to adjust your commute to afford yourself some walking time in the morning or evening. Parking a twenty-minute walk away from your office may seem silly at first, but this simple change helps you burn an extra five hundred calories per week.

All of this has to do with how the physical environment in your neighborhood surroundings influences you. So how can you turn the tables on this and exert some influence yourself? The best way is to engage your social connections, opening their eyes to the problem. This will help you build a team to confront and overcome these challenges.

So if your neighborhood physical environment is less than conducive to walking, why not apply a solution we discussed in an earlier chapter? Getting together with your neighbors to establish a safe walking trail may be one option. This may also be a way to increase security for you and those in your immediate community, if that is a concern in your area.

The strategy we talked about earlier in which you park a twenty-minute walk away from your office may be even more effective if you are part of a carpool. The encouragement you offer and receive from your fellow commuters could be just what you need to keep the healthy adjustment to your physical environment going.

How Technology and Social Media Can Help You Reshape Your Physical Environment

All of those gadgets, gizmos, and mobile widgets on your personal device aren't just for keeping up with your work and personal e-mail. New apps can turn your smartphone and tablet into formidable tools to help you manage your weight—and they also have the benefit of keeping you in close contact with your social structure for motivation and support. One popular option is MyFitnessPal, which includes a calorie counter and diet tracker. Another app, called Gym Pact, adds an incentive to keeping your gym routine going. You join a community in which everyone pledges how many days they will work out in a given month. Miss your goal and you lose money (!!!). Hit it, and you recover your bet, along with the money forfeited by users who did not meet their exercise goals.

As for Jack, his first BlackBerry was the bit of technology he needed to escape the physical environment of his office.

"Before all this happened I bought a Bowflex that I was going

Remember, much of the change that lies within our power is made easier when we use our influence with others to tackle potential problems.

Turning the Tables on Your Physical Environment

We opened this chapter by meeting Jack, who by all accounts was in an unusually difficult situation with regard to his physical environment.

to leave in my office," he says. "Once I got the BlackBerry and could actually check my e-mail outside of the office, I thought, 'I'm never going to be in the office ever again.'" Now he can respond to e-mails while taking a brisk walk through the park instead of being tied to a chair (as long as he keeps an eye on where he is going, that is).

A BlackBerry or iPhone isn't the only technological tool you may find handy when changing your physical environment. For many, social media platforms like Facebook, Twitter, and Foursquare make it possible to tap into social networks and even "check in" at healthy locations—effectively leveraging social pressure toward a healthier lifestyle.

Meanwhile, a host of new gadgets include pedometers that count the steps you take in a day. Fitbit, one of the most popular of these options, tracks your steps and feeds the information into your computer via Bluetooth so you can track your progress. You may be surprised to discover how a simple tool like this can encourage you to make the most of your daily physical environment—essentially "improving your score" every time you take the far parking space in the company lot rather than the one right next to the door, or take the stairs instead of the elevator. These gadgets can even lead to healthy competition within your social network: Vying against your friends to see who can take the most steps in a day can quickly turn into a fun and healthy activity for all involved.

Can You Take Your Positive Physical Environment with You?

Many Americans are almost constantly on the road for their work. As anyone who has ever traveled for work knows, a waistline-friendly physical environment can be difficult to carve out between airport terminals, hotel suites, and boardrooms.

So what can you do about your physical environment if you are in a hotel with no gym or fitness amenities, no pool, and no runner-friendly routes in the surrounding area?

The trick is to improvise. The world is your gym, even if you are on the go. And some inexpensive products may help. For example, you may want to consider packing some fitness bands in your luggage. You can get them cheap—affordable models are $10 to $20—and they won't take up much room in your bag. Plus, they will offer enough resistance for you to get a decent twenty- to thirty-minute workout at the start of your day.

Pushup grips are another solution. These pack easily and will give you a bit more bang for your buck for a quick morning or evening workout when you are on the road. Like fitness bands, these will set you back only about 20 bucks max.

These are small steps, to say the least, but they might be just the thing you need to nudge the physical environment of your hotel room (or layover terminal) into a healthier configuration.

We also detailed the various adjustments he made to his routine that improved how he interacted with this challenging backdrop to his day-to-day life.

We did not tell you a couple of things, however. One is that Jack readily admits he is not perfect in sticking to the tips that have helped him so dramatically thus far. Some days, he says, his surroundings and schedule make exercise impossible and eating healthily extremely difficult.

Improving the Physical Environment of Your Workplace

If you are currently employed, it's likely you spend eight hours or more per day in your workplace. That is eight or so hours every day to steep in the physical environment there, whether it is healthy or not. Unfortunately, we are finding out that these environments seem to be getting less and less healthy for our waistlines as time goes by.

Consider a recent study by Tim Church, MD, MPH, PhD, of Louisiana State University, and his colleagues. Using the famous National Health and Nutrition Examination Survey data from the US Centers for Disease Control and Prevention, they found that daily occupation-related energy expenditure has decreased by more than one hundred calories over the past fifty years.[8]

Simply put, we are expending fewer calories on average in the workplace than our parents did, and these extra calories can lead to expanding waistlines. This is no small impact. In their report, Dr. Church and his colleagues attributed a "significant portion of the increase in mean US body weights for women and men" to decreased calorie burn in the workplace, likely a result of the physical environment. Reinforcing this notion is a Johns Hopkins study led by Jeremy Steeves, PhD, MPH, which demonstrated that those in an occupation with high activity levels had about 37 percent less chance of abdominal obesity than those in low-activity occupations, even when both groups were sedentary outside of work.[9]

So what can you do to tip the scales back in your favor? One way is to think simple when it comes to the physical environment of your office: Take stairs instead of elevators and try to make the most of tasks that allow you to get up and walk around rather than remain in a chair all day.

The other way is to talk with your colleagues as well as human resources, to see what you can do as a team to improve the physical environment of your office. Might it be possible to add a simple walking trail in an area around or near your office? Would a bicycle storage room help encourage everyone in your office to take their bikes to work more often? Maybe it is even possible to get the ball rolling on an office gym. Spread your influence, explore all the options, and see what you can do to work together to get it done.

The other is that Jack's efforts with regard to his physical environment led to healthy changes in other areas of his life, too. Today, despite his demanding schedule, he is a triathlete who regularly competes in Ironman competitions.

Get on Your Bike: Your Neighborhood's "Bikeability"

In cultures around the world—most notably in some European and Asian cities—the bicycle is widely accepted as a mode of transportation. In these cities, bicycling from place to place has become the norm. The overall layout of streets and amenities in these areas is remarkably conducive to riding a bicycle—in many cases, the infrastructure itself has been specifically designed to be friendly toward bicyclers.

An interesting example is the city of Amsterdam in the Netherlands. Here, bicycles are ubiquitous, which should be immediately clear to anyone who has crossed the Prins Hendrikkade outside of Amsterdam's Centraal Station at rush hour. As a result, transportation by bicycle has become a norm here that opens the door to myriad fringe benefits. Commuting and exercise become one and the same. You can carry fewer groceries in a bicycle basket than you can in a car trunk, so daily trips to the market mean fresh, nutritious foods are prioritized over packaged fare. All of this represents how the physical environment can impact your health.

There are neighborhoods and communities in the United States and Canada, too, in which riding a bicycle from place to place is a convenient, safe, and healthy alternative to sitting behind the wheel of your car. In fact, the group behind the aforementioned Walk Score in collaboration with Canadian professors Meghan Winters, PhD, of Simon Fraser University and Michael Brauer, ScD, and Kay Teschke, PhD, of the University of British Columbia have devised a scoring system to assess the bikeability of various US and Canadian metropolitan areas. Called (predictably enough) Bike

"Feeling good is a pretty strong drug," Jack laughs. "Waking up in the morning and not having your lower back hurting—that's a strong thing. There's a lot to be said for exercising and staying healthy, not just to live longer but to live better. It can turn into an addiction."

Score, it takes into account four components related to the ease with which inhabitants can use their bicycles as a primary mode of conveyance: the presence of designated bicycle lanes, the presence of hills, the accessibility of various amenities by bicycle, and the degree to which bicycle commuting is a norm—a measure the architects of this score term "mode share."

According to this formula, if you are hoping to start pedaling to work and other places, you're pretty fortunate if you happen to live in Minneapolis, Portland (Oregon, not Maine), or San Francisco.[10]

Of course, your community's Bike Score is just one factor in using your bicycle for commuting purposes. Inclement weather, for example, or lack of a place to safely store your bicycle at home or at work are just a couple of the challenges you may face. But looking to your social networks—your co-workers or your circle of friends—could help overcome some of these problems. Starting a bicycling group among your social contacts or within your community may make it easier to use your influence to change some of these obstacles. If you happen to live in a condo building in the city, perhaps getting a few of your fellow tenants interested in bicycling will help you convince the condo board to consider a secure storage area for bicycles in your building. Or if you are a suburb dweller, starting a group like this may make on-the-road outings a safer, more regular routine among you and your neighbors. Spread your influence far enough, and you may even be able to collect a group large enough to influence your local government to institute more bike paths and trails. Imagine for a moment how many lives and routines in your community could be changed!

The point is, as with so many of the other things we have discussed, you will meet obstacles in your efforts to create new norms for yourself and others. But many of the obstacles may be surmountable if you leverage your influence in various social networks.

Thinfluence Action Plan: Your Physical Environment

In this chapter we have explored the myriad factors in your physical environment that affect your weight, as well as the steps you can take to make simple changes that can help you exert more control over your weight. Now we will use the system we have established in previous chapters to take a closer look at your particular situation.

ANALYZE

1. How would you describe the physical environment within your home?

   A. The physical layout of my home is not conducive to healthy food choices or healthy activities. My current living arrangement either does not have the space for an area devoted to regular meals or the areas that are intended for dining are not currently used for this. Additionally, my kitchen setup is far from optimal to help me reach for the healthiest options first. As for the rest of my home, candy bowls or unhealthy snacks are conveniently placed in numerous areas. I have TVs in more than one room, and the areas for TV watching are also used for eating and snacking.

   B. The physical environment in my home definitely has one or two unhealthy aspects. It may be a dining area conveniently within viewing distance of a TV, or it could be that clutter in the kitchen makes it difficult to prepare healthy foods on a regular basis.

   C. In the course of my "home inspection," I can find very little in my immediate physical environment that might support an unhealthy routine. TV areas, if they exist in my home, are far from the areas where meals are enjoyed. It is easy to prepare healthy meals in my home, and a yard or other outdoor area can be used for exercise and healthy hobbies.

2. Scout out your neighborhood. What do you see with regard to the physical environment?

A. The prospect of taking a leisurely walk in my neighborhood is, frankly, a bit frightening. Few, if any, green spaces like parks are nearby. No sidewalk is in sight. And other factors, such as traffic or a high crime rate in the area, further discourage physical activity outdoors.

B. After reading this chapter, I can pick out at least one or two features of my neighborhood that would support healthy activities—a well-maintained sidewalk, for example, or a neighborhood park.

C. My neighborhood is a paradise for outdoor physical activities like walking, jogging, and bicycling. Numerous, well-used green spaces are nearby, and many in the neighborhood flock to these community resources.

3. Now look at your community as a whole. What are the features of the physical environment within your greater community?

A. The community in which I live is sprawling, and most everyone lives in areas that require a car to get back and forth from work every day. There are no bicycle lanes, and mass transit options are either inconvenient or absent altogether. On most days, the weather or pollution levels make being outdoors difficult.

B. While finding a car-free approach to my commute might be a challenge in my community, I have to admit that it would not be impossible. Some other features within my community encourage physical activity, such as a conveniently situated walking track or some other common amenity.

C. The community in which I live is very conducive to an active lifestyle. In many cases, the places where people work are convenient to residential areas, and roads are bicycle friendly. Mass transit options are also plentiful, making it possible to live conveniently without using a car. My community has green spaces galore.

ACT

Take a look at your responses to the questions. What do you see?

◊ **Mostly As:** Though it may seem that the odds are stacked against you in terms of your physical environment, don't despair—some relatively simple changes will likely help you make the best of your surroundings. Start in your home: Make sure your dining area, kitchen, and all other areas are optimized for healthy behaviors. Once you have done this, you can start looking at your neighborhood and community. See if you can devise a way to conduct your daily routine that incorporates a healthy dose of passive activity. Every additional twenty steps you can add to your routine, every staircase you can take instead of an elevator—each of these things, if you turn it into a habit, can add up to weight loss.

◊ **Mostly Bs:** It sounds like your physical surroundings offer some opportunities for increasing your daily activity level. While they may not be right in front of you, it is up to you to test-drive a few possibilities to see how you can take advantage of what is available. Try taking some of the simple steps we recommended in this chapter—switching up your commute to incorporate a bit more walking, or even seeing if it is possible to get back and forth from your place of work without using a car at all. Better yet, get your friends and family in on these changes. The more people you can influence to tackle these challenges, the better your chances of success.

◊ **Mostly Cs:** Congratulations! It sounds like your physical environment is ideal for weight-friendly living. But are you taking full advantage of what is offered? Make a list of the opportunities that your surroundings present for additional physical activity, pick one or two of these opportunities to start with, and make them part of your daily routine. A bit of effort in the right direction will be rewarded.

In addition to the strategies above, you can try some simple things in your daily routine that carry big dividends toward getting to a healthy weight:

◊ If there is a park, walking trail, or other outdoor area near your home that you do not frequently visit, make it a point to incorporate walking or exercise time there into your weekly routine. To reinforce this routine, bring in your family members or neighborhood acquaintances. Together you can make full use of this neighborhood resource. And it's free!

◊ Explore starting a family or community garden. This not only will provide fresh vegetables and other food choices, but will also be a good way to incorporate a bit more physical activity into your routine.

◊ Make physical activity a game by keeping score based on how much physical activity you get in the course of your day. This is where a pedometer or Fitbit can come in especially handy. Once you see how many steps you take in a day, you can keep pushing the envelope to achieve your personal best. This works even better if you can bring others into the game or even share your personal best over a social media network. Turning daily physical activity into a competition is a great way to keep yourself motivated and influence others, too!

INFLUENCE

One important thing to remember about nearly any physical environment you encounter is that you are not in it alone. Your family, your neighbors, your co-workers—all of them have something to gain (or weight to lose) from improving their interactions with their physical environment. To get the ball rolling, consider some incentives you can use to get them on your side:

◊ Better health and weight control thanks to more regular physical activity

◊ Financial incentives through savings on gasoline thanks to alternative transportation

◊ Strengthened community relationships and support

As we have discussed, the key is finding those around you whom you can influence and motivate. On your own, changing your physical environment (or making the most of what you have available) may seem like an insurmountable challenge. But with motivation and support from others, you may find some simple solutions you would not have come up with on your own.

Physical Environment Solutions: Try It Today!

While some aspects of changing your physical environment may seem daunting, take heart: You can incorporate some things into your daily routine immediately. Consider the following simple steps:

◊ When you are watching television, get up and march in place or do some deep knee bends while the commercials are running. It may feel silly at first. But consider for a moment that each half hour of television programming contains seven to ten minutes of commercials, and it quickly becomes clear that sticking to this simple rule can burn some serious calories. And you won't have to miss your favorite shows!

◊ Try planning a "green space treasure hunt" in your neighborhood, in which you aim to find at least three good places to get outdoor exercise near your home. Better yet, spread the idea around your social connections to start up some friendly competition to find the best spots.

◊ Establish "no eating" zones in your home. These could be areas close to the television and other distractions. It's a simple and easily enforceable rule—and it could improve your whole family's health and weight in the long run.

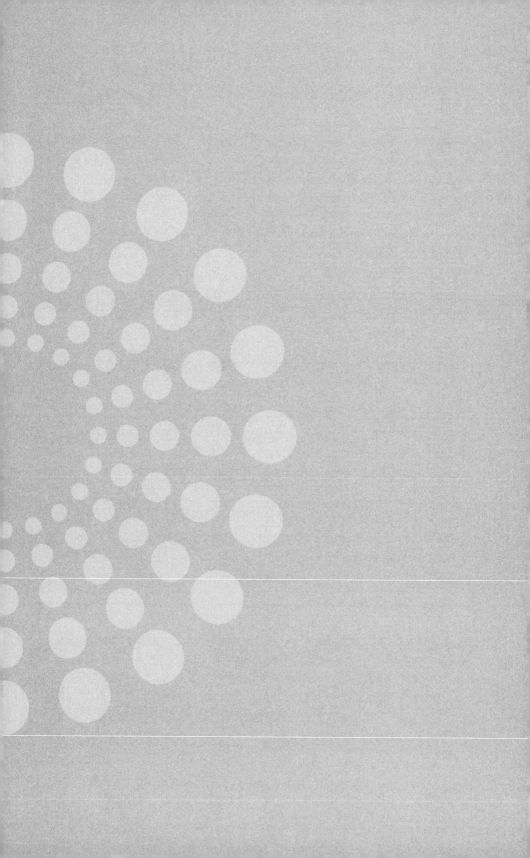

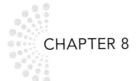

Your Media "Diet": The Impact of Information and Advertising

You wake up in the morning to the sound of your clock radio. In the time it takes you to switch off the alarm, you hear part of a tantalizing ad about a hot sausage and egg muffin available at the nearby drive-thru restaurant.

Once you towel off from the shower and brush your teeth, you switch on the television and watch it out of the corner of your eye as you get dressed. The morning news and entertainment show is featuring a piece on the newest trend diet to take the country by storm . . . followed by a segment on a hamburger that uses glazed doughnuts instead of a bun. In between news segments, you see an ad for a new product that can help you twist, twist, twist away the pounds at your midsection. This advertisement is followed by another that spotlights a new line of cheese-infused entrées at a popular restaurant chain. (Did they just say "Cheese-fest"? Don't know what that means, but it sounds pretty tempting. . . .)

You hop into your car and turn on the radio for the commute, where you hear again about that sausage and egg muffin. Coincidentally, it seems, you pass a billboard indicating that the drive-thru offering this breakfast item is right on your way to the office. You need a hot coffee anyway, and you have a couple of bucks in your wallet—what's the harm? You pull into the drive-thru, where you are greeted by a friendly voice from the menu board speaker.

You get to your office and carry your coffee with you as you enter the doors—you already polished off that sausage muffin in the car. You settle in at your cubicle, taking a few brief breaks throughout the morning to surf the Web for a few seconds at a time. As you browse, you notice some soft drink ads, as well as a couple for a popular brand of salty corn snacks. Hey, was that a coupon? *Need to remember that for later,* you think to yourself.

It's lunchtime, and a few of your colleagues are heading out for a bite. Inviting you to come along, they ask if you have any suggestions. You mention that you heard something about a Cheese-fest and that it also involved unlimited breadsticks. Your suggestion is wholeheartedly approved by the group, and you head out for a filling and savory meal.

You return to the office after lunch, and the afternoon is loaded with meetings and deadlines. About midafternoon, you realize that you might have to stay at the office an hour or so later, which means a late dinner. Not wanting to "run out of gas" later on, you head to the vending machines, where you pick up a bag of a popular brand of salty corn snacks and a can of cola.

The day ends late, but not quite as late as you had expected. On your way out of work, you glance at the television to see one of your favorite singing competitions, sponsored by a major soft drink company.

On your way home, you listen again to the radio. You don't know what to have for dinner yet, but ever since you saw that fried chicken ad, you can't seem to get it out of your mind. You stop by the drive-thru on the way home and pick up a fried chicken meal. *Just this time this week,* you rationalize to yourself. *It was a busy day at work.*

Back in your house, you flip on the TV as you prepare to eat. A commercial for an herbal pill promises to zap away the fat at your midsection. A computer animation shows this process at work, and a bikini-wearing model stands proudly next to a giant poster of what she looked like "before." Some fine print at the bottom of the screen says something about results not being typical and how the FDA has not evaluated . . . wait, we're on to the next commercial.

You sit down on the sofa after dinner to watch your favorite show, which every week scours restaurants from state to state in search of the ten most decadent burgers in the country. You see the ad for the new exercise device again—the one where you can simply twist, twist, twist your way to a beach-ready body. *It's hard not to be skeptical*, you think to yourself. But looking down at the pounds around your midsection, you begin to wonder if it might not be worth a shot. After all, there is a thirty-day money-back guarantee. And since your New Year's resolution to make healthier choices for your weight does not seem to be panning out as you had hoped, you could use all the help you can get.

That's when you suddenly experience a familiar, frustrating feeling. You think back over your choices during the day. What on earth, you wonder, might be causing you to make so many decisions that keep you at an unhealthy weight?

How the Media Influences Your Weight Decisions

The example of a typical day described here may or may not fit your personal experience. But it is likely that at least part of it sounds familiar to you. Maybe you are a stay-at-home parent who doesn't listen to the radio on a regular basis but watches a fair amount of television. Or perhaps you are a shift worker who is seldom awake for the morning television shows but spends a considerable amount of time surfing the Internet in your free time.

No matter what your day looks like, one thing all of us have in common is that we are continually confronted with commercials, entertainment, advertisements, and other forms of marketing. And many of these messages either directly or indirectly push products or services that have some kind of effect on decisions that relate to our weight.

This, of course, should come as little surprise. We are all aware on some level that advertisements are (1) intended to sell us something and

(2) designed to make us desire that thing enough to buy it. In short, it is easy to tell ourselves that we understand what is going on here.

Yet simply understanding how media messages work doesn't make us immune to them any more than understanding the weather forecast keeps us dry. Media advertising and marketing work, regardless of whether the messages help or hurt your efforts to achieve or maintain a healthy weight.

Just as we have described in previous chapters how important it is to be aware of the influences of your social and physical surroundings, so, too, is it important to take a mindful approach to the messages you are exposed to every single day. The ability to really distinguish the messages that are good for your weight from the ones that are harmful is becoming more necessary with each passing decade—especially considering that we are exposed to a growing array of media that carry messages both hidden and overt about weight and health. Research is beginning to reveal how advertisements and other media messages can affect our weight,[1,2,3] and unfortunately there are more than enough negative, unhealthy messages to go around. Whether it is a celebrity TV chef whose calorie-laden dishes normalize unhealthy eating, fast-food advertisements that hold appeal for children, or the promotion of over-the-counter weight loss products that promise more than they deliver, it appears that few of us are not somehow targeted.

In this chapter, we will look at the messages that you—along with millions of other American adults, adolescents, and children—receive through advertisements and other media about weight loss and food choices. Most important, we will explore how we, as consumers, can empower ourselves and our loved ones to separate fact from fiction in these messages, so you can make healthier choices and influence others to do so as well.

It is our hope that by better recognizing these messages and dealing with them appropriately, you and your loved ones can adjust your "media diet" and leverage the power of your relationships to reinforce healthier consumption of media messages.

Media and Your Mass: The Influence of Advertisements

We often hear that we are "bombarded" by messages in the media about our weight and our health. Bombardment is an apt analogy—many of these messages explode into our field of attention so overtly, they constitute an assault on our senses. However, many of the messages directed at us through the media are far more subtle, though they may have no less of an effect on the choices we make.

Messages as close as your TV remote or radio dial often come in the form of commercial advertisements for foods that are less than healthy, to say the least. While we know that Americans are exposed to a staggering amount of this information, it is hard to say exactly how many of these ads we are exposed to on a regular basis. Researchers have, however, looked closely at one segment of the population in terms of advertisement exposure: children.

Why children? The conventional wisdom about kids and teens is that they are voracious consumers of media—and in this case, science reveals that the conventional wisdom is true. In many ways, we can look at kids and teens as canaries in the coal mine regarding the effects of messages broadcasted in our cars, our homes, and over the Internet. To put a number on this consumption, a recent study published in the journal *Pediatrics* showed that children and teenagers spend, on average, more than seven hours every day using media such as television, computers, and cell phones.[4]

What messages are young people receiving through these devices? Researchers at the Kaiser Family Foundation sought to answer this question when they conducted the largest study of its kind to date on television watching in children and teens.[5] They found that the amount of television watching—and with it, exposure to advertisements for food—varied among age groups. But one thing held true among each of these age groups: The sheer number of ads to which adolescents and teens are exposed every year is huge, no matter their age. They determined, for example, that children ages eight to twelve watched an average of twenty-one food ads per day on TV. This translates to more than 7,600 food ads per year in this age group, the equivalent of spending more than two twenty-four-hour days perched in front of the TV, watching these commercials. The Kaiser researchers found that teens ages thirteen to seventeen were exposed, on average, to slightly fewer of these ads, though these teens still saw, on average, seventeen food advertisements per day. That's more than six thousand ads per year or about forty straight hours' worth of food advertisements.

What do these advertisements tell our kids? The Kaiser researchers found that 15 percent of them portrayed a healthy lifestyle, regardless of how healthy the product itself happened to be. Twenty-two percent included what the researchers termed a disclaimer, such as "part of a balanced diet" or "part of a healthy breakfast." Other ads were more direct: 13 percent included at least one specific health claim. As far as enticement to buy (or get their parents to buy) the product, 11 percent of the advertisements featured a children's television or movie character, and 7 percent used a contest or sweepstakes.

But is exposure to these messages problematic in and of itself? Not necessarily. One could imagine, for example, that ads for whole grain products or fruits and vegetables might be a good thing. However, the researchers looked into this, too. They found that of all the ads to which kids were exposed, 34 percent—more than a third—were for candy and snacks. Roughly 28 percent were for cereal, and 10 percent were for fast food. Of the remaining quarter of food ads watched by kids and teens, 4 percent were for dairy products. One percent of these ads were for fruit juices. Virtually none were for fruits or vegetables.

What could rightfully be seen as the antidote to these messages— public service announcements, or PSAs, for healthy food or exercise—were at one time a staple of Saturday morning television (Schoolhouse Rock? . . . Anyone?). But it seems that such PSAs are a dying breed in today's television environment; kids ages eight to twelve see on average just one of these PSAs every two to three days, for a total of one hour and fifteen minutes of these messages each year. Teens see even fewer of these PSAs; they are exposed to an average of forty-seven PSAs for fitness and nutritious food choices per year, just twenty-five minutes of such content.

These and other reports likely led the American Academy of Pediatrics in 2011 to push Congress to institute a ban on junk food ads during children's TV shows.

For fairly obvious reasons, far less research has gone into the messages adults get from advertisements. As adults, we imagine ourselves to be less vulnerable to such messages, as well as far more entitled to a certain degree of freedom in choosing what to see and how to eat or exercise.

Yet our sense of security may be false if we believe that, as adults, we are somehow impervious to the influence of media on our health and weight. Consider Nielsen findings that Americans, on average, watch nearly thirty-five hours of television every week. That's about five hours a day and nearly ten hours per week more TV than is watched by children ages two to eleven. Much of the advertising and marketing to which we are exposed is similar to what our kids are exposed to—fast food, sugary drinks, and indulgent food. After all, a very lucrative industry has risen around such products.

Meanwhile, the humble asparagus spear hardly merits a mention in the daytime TV schedule, much less during prime time. Pity the green leafy vegetables, the pinto beans, and the carrots as well. These items— arguably among the healthiest things we could be putting in our refrigerators and on our dinner tables—have little or no brand recognition. But ask someone what their favorite soda or candy bar is, and they are likely to have an answer.

All of this is because the food industry spends massive amounts on marketing research that examines human behavior and neuroscience. This research is to determine what messages sell best, and constant competition between food manufacturers means that advertisers are getting better and better at designing messages with each passing year.

So if you doubt that these messages exert considerable influence when we make choices affecting our weight, consider this question: Would it make any sense whatsoever for companies to pour millions, even billions, of dollars into sharpening and targeting their messages if they did *not* work?

Even for those of us who feel—correctly or not—that we are somehow not influenced by advertisements, exposure to various media can still affect our health decisions in many ways. And be warned: Not all of them are as overt as a cartoon bear selling us sweetened cereal.

Mixed Messages about Food and Weight

Looking beyond advertisements, other types of media messages can influence our eating and exercise behaviors; these messages often "fly under our radar." A number of them fall into a category we will call The Unhealthiest "Healthy" Messages You'll Hear.

Some are "magic bullet" messages concerning weight loss or exercise. The promises are almost too tempting to ignore. As a result, the companies behind the bevy of products that promise a better bikini body, a more muscled torso, or less fat around our bellies have managed to turn our hopes into a highly profitable industry. The success of such ads is largely driven by customer testimonials—and the stories are usually so dramatic, it is easy to miss the "results not typical" fine print at the bottom of the screen.

Progress has been made in reining in some of these advertisements, particularly those involving bogus weight loss pills and formulas. In fact, in the last decade regulators became more active in controlling ads for these gimmicky products, beginning with the Federal Trade Commission, which in 2002 released its first report on weight loss advertising. But ads for over-the-counter weight loss products that make big promises based on little proof are still pervasive. In 2011, researchers from Cornell and Carnegie Mellon Universities found that about one in ten men and women who were exposed to ads for these products actually purchased and tried them.[6] And while a small percentage of them may have achieved the atypical results they were promised, others were likely left feeling more than a bit disappointed—and still struggling with the same weight issues that led them to buy the advertised product in the first place.

Advertisements relating to quick or easy weight loss span a broad range of product categories. What products are we talking about, specifically? We're not going to name names . . . but they tend to fall largely into the following categories.

Weight loss supplements: Take a pill a day, do nothing else, and watch the pounds melt away. What could be easier? Never mind that the bottle says these products "have not been evaluated by the Food and Drug Administration" and are "not intended to diagnose, treat, cure, or prevent any disease or health condition."

"Spot-reducing" exercise equipment: Just ten minutes a day is all you need to crunch, crunch, crunch your way to a flat, toned tummy. Or to get rid of saddlebags, cellulite, etc. All for anywhere from $29.95 to several hundred dollars. For the doubters out there, the before-and-after testimonials show the incredible payoff of using the product in question— accompanied, of course, by the short disclaimer "results not typical."

Gimmicky diets: Who hasn't heard by now of the grapefruit diet, the cabbage soup diet, or any one of a number of other juice or "negative-calorie" food regimens that claim thirty-day results? In most cases, these diets attempt to take the proven advice of cutting back on calories and turn it on its head in some way. Unfortunately, for most of these diets, the only thing you lose in the end is the illusion that they actually work.

"Extreme" fitness DVDs: This one's a little tough. Unlike the options listed above, these involve an actual commitment of time and sweat. And unlike the other categories, if you stick with the recommended regimens, you will see results. However, where these products fall short is sustainability. Sure, for a small percentage of people, these programs will represent a true, lasting lifestyle change. But for everyone else, completing the prescribed duration of thirty days to three months leaves you at risk of slipping back into old habits and routines. Fail to keep up or sustain an injury, and you are back to square one . . . or worse.

At best, many of these magic bullet approaches simply lead to disappointment. At worst, they can feed the very weight problems they purport to solve. Recently one of Malissa's patients, whose goal was to lose thirty pounds, admitted that she had been skipping from fad diet to fad diet but had hit a wall with regard to her weight loss. When Malissa asked her if she was familiar with Walter's Healthy Eating Plate—which limits

The Rise of "Food Porn"

In 1963, public television audiences were introduced to what would eventually become a decades-long phenomenon. On February 11 of that year, an American chef and author named Julia Child presented the first episode of *The French Chef.* It was not the first time a cooking show had aired on television, but it was one of the most memorable forays into the idea of cooking and cuisine as entertainment. In the years that followed, Child would become a household name.

Fast-forward fifty years, and it is nothing short of amazing to see how far food entertainment has come. Cooking shows and programs about food pervade the airwaves. Many cable subscribers enjoy access to not one, but two channels devoted to food preparation and enjoyment—the Food Network and the Cooking Channel. A number of the programs on these channels celebrate the preparation of healthy meals from whole, fresh ingredients, often in conjunction with a healthy lifestyle. On the other end of the spectrum are programs that showcase greasy diner food served in gargantuan portions, fat- and cholesterol-laden southern "comfort food," and, of course, cupcakes by the baker's dozen.

In the middle are a broad range of offerings: some healthy, some not so much. But no matter the cuisine, the very existence of such networks makes one thing exceedingly clear: We are a culture obsessed with food. This conclusion rings even more true online, where innumerable "foodie" carbohydrates to whole grains that should take up no more than one-fourth of the plate—the woman was aghast. She said that according to the diets she had been following, it was normal for her plate to be 75 percent occupied by carbs. Malissa explained to her that the concept of a "diet" as a quick and painless cure actually leads to disappointment and lack of success, not to mention increased weight gain down the road.

blogs and Web sites present an even wider range of options for us to seek out or try to make ourselves—from vegan, low-carb mini-meals to the state-fair-inspired deep-fried sticks of butter.

We should not be surprised, then, that the slick, glamorous, irresistible, and exotic presentation of many of these foods has earned its own widely recognized moniker. It's a term you may have heard yourself: food porn.

The food porn movement has arguably stoked our culture's already widespread obsession with tasty food, and it has had its fair share of champions. One particularly well-known personality, renowned for such crowd-pleasers as "fried butter balls" (butter mixed with cream cheese, breaded, and fried in peanut oil) and "lasagna soup," has received equal measures of criticism and praise for her creations. That was until 2012, when her diagnosis of type 2 diabetes led her to retool many of her recipes—and to become a paid spokesperson for a major pharmaceutical company marketing a diabetes management program.

How should we confront this cultural obsession with food, both individually and within our social circles? It's a complex question with no single, simple answer. Perhaps the most important step, though, is to remain mindful of the influence of the food porn culture. Whether we are watching an hourlong pork belly cooking competition between two master chefs, a show that teaches us how to prepare a light and delightful Mediterranean salad, or a tutorial on the proper way to deep-fry a stick of butter, the most important thing to keep in mind is that these media messages carry a heavy influence. It's okay to be entertained . . . as long as you are ready to pinch yourself before heading to your own pantry or kitchen.

The bottom line is that much of the marketing and advertising we see treats satisfactory weight as a valuable commodity. Bear this in mind the next time you see an advertisement for a product that promises to help you drop the pounds, selectively burn the fat around your midsection, or

TV Watching and Your Health: What Research Shows

In this chapter, we explore the idea of the media content we consume and how it may affect our weight, and we look at some of the more recent research into this issue. But it is interesting to note that researchers have been studying this relationship for years—and what they have found draws a clear line between TV time and your weight.

Back in 1996, Walter and his colleagues at Harvard examined the impact of TV time on the chances of being overweight.[7] The result was one of the early studies on the matter, and it used information gathered through the Health Professionals Follow-Up Study. This study looked at adult men and compared their TV-watching habits to their odds of being overweight. It found that men who watched forty-one or more hours of television or videos per week were more than four times as likely to

be overweight as men watching no more than one hour per week.

It was a tantalizing finding, and one that Walter and his colleagues would continue to explore. Further analysis of the data from the study showed than TV watching was related not only to the risk of being overweight, but also to an increase in markers in the blood tied to the risk of heart disease. Other research has demonstrated similar links to diabetes risk.[8]

All of this tells us that a link appears to exist between excess television consumption and various weight- and heart-related ills. True, some of these may have to do with the actual sedentary act of sitting on the couch for that sitcom marathon. However, the evidence shows that the way the messages we get through television influence our diets and actions is also to blame.

achieve other desirable traits associated with weight loss. These messages may have the veneer of health, but they could end up letting you down in the long run.

Online Media: What It's Telling You

Land grab. It's a term that evokes images of the US expansion in the 1800s. Today something very similar is happening, except that the plots of "land" are marketing and advertising opportunities online. In both cases, a sudden increase in territory and possibilities led to a rush to stake claims. Likewise both events presented situations that appeared to outstrip the laws and guidelines put into place to keep all of us out of harm's way.

Sure, there are some differences—for example, there were arguably fewer funny cat pictures circulating back then. But today's online marketing and advertising landscape begins to seem an awful lot like the Wild West when you really sit down and look at it. Indeed, as the Internet, social media, and other new and emerging forms of communication have become more intertwined with our lives, a wave of new research has uncovered some of the effects that media and advertising have on many of the choices that affect our weight. In short, the picture is not pretty.

To study food marketing trends online, researchers at the Rudd Center for Food Policy and Obesity at Yale University looked closely at how food marketers promote their products and brands through social media platforms such as Facebook, Twitter, and YouTube.[9] They found that not only did many major food brands maintain profiles, accounts, and channels on these platforms, but in many cases their corporate presences were among the most popular out there. On Facebook, for example, numerous food brands' profiles fell into the top twenty in

Taking Health News Headlines with a Grain of Salt

As much as Dan hates to admit it, at times the news media does not get the message exactly right when it comes to healthy, responsible decisions for weight loss and weight maintenance. Much of this has to do with the reporting of "new" findings about dieting and weight loss in newspapers and on TV.

For example, is it really true, according to some 2012 reports by major news media outlets, that the key to staying slim is eating chocolate? Or, according to another wave of 2012 reports, that red wine blocks fat cell formation, thus potentially cutting your risk of obesity?

The writers of these articles come by these delightfully counterintuitive headlines honestly; the research they invoke was legitimate, published in prominent, peer-reviewed scientific journals. And yet they fail to convey the very important caveats included in the studies themselves—that the benefits were seen only when consumption was kept to a moderate amount, or that factors other than the chemicals in chocolate and wine might be the real reasons for the health benefits. Even so, these headlines unfortunately may have influenced some people to believe that the key to getting to a healthier weight is to eat a lot more chocolate or drink a lot more red wine.

Nobody in their right mind would jump to these conclusions if it were all up to common sense; chocolate, after all, can come in many delicious forms, many of which come packed with empty calories. Likewise, red wine packs about 150 calories into a six-ounce glass—likely more calories than can be staved off by the ingredients that some research suggests may have a small positive effect in weight maintenance.[10]

These caveats are routinely included in the stories and reports of responsible health and medical journalists. Even then, it is easy to see how the general public may be quick to believe, from the headlines they read, that these counterintuitive messages are the norm rather than the exception in terms of healthy weight behaviors. All too often, this is far from the case.

terms of popularity. The most popular profile of all the brands? Coca-Cola, with more than twenty-four million "fans" as of September 2011.

The researchers acknowledge that it is, as yet, difficult to pin down exactly how much it means to food manufacturers to be popular on Facebook and in other social media forums. But given the resources going into efforts to fill the online space, it is safe to assume that opportunities for advertisers to reach and influence an increasingly connected consumer base are potentially lucrative.

Helping Kids Become Healthier Consumers of Media

Given the steady rise in unhealthy weight in children, some researchers in the field of childhood obesity have come up with interventions to help curb the problem—and more than a few have focused on media consumption.[11] Planet Health was a Harvard School of Public Health program conducted in about twenty schools in Massachusetts in the late 1990s. The program looked at a number of factors believed to contribute to unhealthy weight in childhood. Among them were insufficient fruit and vegetable intake, consumption of high-fat foods, and a general lack of sufficient physical activity. However, another pillar of the program involved limiting television viewing among these children.

The outcomes of Planet Health showed that the program successfully reduced TV time by about half an hour a day for the kids who participated. These children's risk of obesity also dropped. The results were especially notable in girls, and in this group especially it could be seen that with each hour of reduction in TV watching, the odds of being obese went down as well.

Children and Unhealthy Media Messages Online

Given the expansion of the Internet, social media platforms like Facebook and Twitter, and a multitude of other electronic forms of communication, it seems obvious that advertisers of less-than-healthy food options for children would view such outlets as a potential boon. Still, many parents may be surprised, even shocked, to learn the extent to which junk food marketing, both subtle and overt, has infiltrated kids' online time.

In 2008, a Federal Trade Commission report estimated that manufacturers paid roughly $1.6 billion to promote foods and beverages, including soda, cereal, and fast food, to kids in 2006. Some nutrition researchers peg this figure as much higher when all is said and done—especially when fast-food companies are included in the mix. In 2010, researchers at Yale compiled the Fast Food FACTS report,[12] a comprehensive look at the ways fast food may be affecting the health of young people, and they found that the fast-food industry in 2009 spent more than $4.2 billion on advertising.

But where are these advertising and marketing dollars going? Some of them are being spent on a phenomenon known as "advergaming." As the name suggests, advergaming involves the creation of fun, addictive online games in which a product somehow features as part of the game. These games are sometimes hosted on Web sites that are not owned by a food brand—sites like Cartoon Network.com and Neopets.com, for example—and that also contain other games not connected to foods advertised to children. Entire sites, however, are owned by major food brands, and many of these sites contain advergaming. In 2006, three University of Minnesota researchers—Kristi Weber, MPH, RD; Mary Story, PhD, RD; and Lisa Harnack, DrPH, RD—examined food and beverage brand Web sites to determine their marketing strategies for young audiences.[13] Their findings were revealing:

"Advergaming" (games in which the advertised product is part of the game) was present on 63 percent of the Web sites. Half or more of the Web sites used cartoon characters (50 percent) or spokescharacters (55 percent), or had a specially designated children's area (58 percent) with a direct link from the home page.

As for social media, it is important to note that most of the major platforms require new users to attest that they are thirteen years of age or older. Even so, it remains clear that social media is a powerful means by which to influence young consumers to buy certain products. The campaigns these brands use harness the latest technology to pick up information about individuals and their choices, predict behaviors and preferences, and target and direct advertisements appropriately. And these marketing strategies are applied to influence children whether or not the products involved are ultimately good or bad for their health.

"Viral forms of marketing are likely to be most effective at influencing adolescent consumers who are more susceptible to peer influence and highly motivated to fit in with their peers," researchers at Yale University's Rudd Center write in their report. "Although skeptical of traditional forms of marketing, through Facebook and other social media, teens and even younger children are becoming unwitting marketers and exponentially extending the reach of companies' advertising campaigns."

In many ways, this new breed of marketing shows what can be done by exploiting much of the same science we reference in this book, but to a different end. Instead of using the knowledge to help consumers improve their own well-being, this approach aims to improve the corporate bottom line. In essence it's two sides of the same coin—but for most of us, one of these sides is much heavier than the other.

Getting a Grip on Media Messages

If you have looked at the Circles of Influence graph lately, you will notice we are venturing pretty far away from the center (page 10). So it probably seems like it is getting more and more difficult for you to exert your own influence in the spheres we are discussing. Appearances, however, can be deceiving.

Ten or fifteen years ago, little could have been done to deal effectively with marketing and advertising that encouraged choices detrimental to your weight. The answer back then was simple: Turn off the TV or radio, fold up the magazine, or find some other way to simply "turn off" your exposure.

Today, however, the Internet—the very venue now being populated with weight-unfriendly marketing messages—may be most conducive to the healthy influences you generate. How can you use social media and the Internet to spread your influence among those with whom you interact? Perhaps for you the answer is to create a Facebook group designed to allow all members to share their healthy recipes or coordinate their physical activities. Those of us with a literary inclination might choose to start a healthy living blog, or at least resolve to tweet to our followers three healthy messages a day. Already countless individuals are doing these very things online. Why not follow them or subscribe to their blogs? As long as you are connected to someone who offers solid, legitimate advice on your weight, you may find that the online realm is a great source of information and inspiration.

In your home, the age-old advice may remain the same: Limit exposure to ads by limiting TV time, and encourage discussions with your family about the messages you receive in magazines and online.

But whatever strategy you choose, know that you are not powerless. You wield influence, and properly applied, that influence can go a long way to helping you achieve and maintain the weight you want—and help those around you to do the same!

Thinfluence Action Plan: Your Media Environment

By the time you've reached the end of this chapter, hopefully you will have developed a better understanding of the media messages that affect your weight and of how you might be able to mitigate their effect on behaviors that influence your weight. Now let's look at how we can use our Thinfluence Action Plan to better understand and deal with our media environment.

ANALYZE

1. How would you rate your "media diet"? In other words, how much time do you spend consuming media messages each day, and how would you describe the messages you're exposed to?

    A. On most days I spend five or more hours watching TV or surfing the Internet for leisure. I admit that I find food porn entertaining, and I notice many advertisements for foods and beverages while I watch or browse online. I can tell that many of the things I see are not terribly healthy, but the images sure are enticing!

    B. I spend between three and five hours engaged in electronic media, and though I don't consider myself a fan of food porn, I do notice quite a few messages on fattening foods and beverages.

    C. On any given day, I spend only one or two hours of my leisure time watching TV and browsing the Internet, and most of what I see does not have much to do with unhealthy food and/or beverages.

2. Be honest—how susceptible do you feel you are to the messages you see and hear regarding fattening foods and beverages? How about advertisements for weight loss products?

A. I am quite susceptible to such messages, and I regularly buy foods that were advertised to me. Additionally, I have ordered at least one weight loss product advertised on TV or online in the past six months.

B. I have my strong days and my weak days. On occasion I will see something on TV or online that is just too tempting to pass up. As far as weight loss products I have seen advertised, I have purchased at least one in the past.

C. I honestly feel I am not susceptible to these media messages. I can't remember the last time I bought a fattening food or beverage based on an advertisement I saw. And I have never purchased a weight loss product I saw advertised on TV or online.

3. How would you describe your use of social media like Facebook and Twitter?

A. My style is usually that of a follower. I primarily like to see what others are interested in or suggesting in terms of products and experiences, but I rarely put messages out that I feel would influence the behaviors of others.

B. My style could be described as a fifty-fifty approach. I like to follow the interests of others, but I also like to put my own influence out there on occasion.

C. I feel that I am an influencer where social media is concerned. I like to share my ideas and influence among my social circles, and I am quick to speak out on things I disagree with.

ACT

Take a look at your answers to the questions. How did your answers turn out?

◊ **Mostly As:** It seems that you are exposed to a pretty decent dose of media messages, and it is likely that many of them influence the choices you make about your diet and lifestyle habits. For you, a good first step may be to set a reasonable limit within your home for television viewing and Internet use—and stick to it. See if you can replace at least some of your television and online time with healthier activities, like family outdoor time or exercise.

◊ **Mostly Bs:** Your media diet isn't half bad, nor is the way it seems to impact your life. However, it is likely that the messages you are exposed to still guide your behavior in ways that affect your weight. It is crucial that you become an expert in scrutinizing the information that comes your way through the TV, online, or from some other source. Once you do this, it may be possible for you to broadcast your own messages—over social media, for example—to help influence others to make healthier media decisions as well.

◊ **Mostly Cs:** It looks like you are less vulnerable to unhealthy media messages than most, which is a good thing. The next question you should be asking yourself is how you influence those close to you—such as your family and friends—to be wise and skeptical consumers of media messages, too.

Of course, this short questionnaire does not capture every aspect of media exposure within your household. Here are a few additional tips that can help you come up with a strategy for you—and your family, if they live with you—to be an intelligent consumer of media:

◊ If you have kids, know this: The American Academy of Pediatrics recommends no more than two hours of screen time each day, but this should be considered a maximum. When determining TV time for your kids, set rules that encourage them to avoid the times when unhealthy children's products are advertised, such as midafternoon and weekend mornings.

◊ Learn how to police what your children see on TV and the sites they are visiting. Learn to recognize the messages they are receiving and talk to them about the difference between what they are seeing and what represents a healthy diet. A good online resource for parents is kidshealth.org. This site features a special section on how TV can affect your child's weight, and it offers tips to help teach good TV habits to your child.

◊ Whether you have kids or not, when you are online, steer clear of Web sites that pitch a product; these usually end in ".com" or another extension that denotes a business. Try instead to focus on ".gov," ".org," or ".edu" Web sites, which tend to be more scientific and valid in their approaches.

INFLUENCE

Because of the surreptitious nature of media influence, you may be surprised by the positive effects of making a few adjustments here and there in how you approach the information and entertainment you consume—and by how those changes can make it easier for you to achieve a better weight. But as always, it helps to have others on your side. Here are some of the benefits you and others can expect with a healthier approach to media habits:

◊ A healthier self image

◊ A more informed and aware approach to media

◊ More meaningful family time

◊ Better instincts when faced with advertisements designed to capitalize on weight insecurities

Share these positive outcomes, and you can influence others, too.

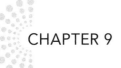

CHAPTER 9

Policy: What Is It? And How Does It Affect Your Weight?

In many ways, looking at the Mississippi Delta county of Holmes is a bit like peering into the future of the country's weight problem.

Already, Holmes County residents live in a state that is, according to statistics from the Centers for Disease Control and Prevention (CDC), one of the most obese in the country. So serious is Mississippi's weight problem that nearly seven out of every ten adults in the state are at an unhealthy weight.

But in Holmes County, the picture is even worse. Consistently it ranks among the worst of all of Mississippi's eighty-two counties in measures of obesity and physical inactivity. In 2011 it was officially the most obese county in the nation, according to CDC figures. It is a place where children as young as three are diagnosed with high blood pressure, and a recent study by a team of US and UK researchers revealed that between 2000 and 2007, this county had the among worst life expectancies in the country.[1]

More than 1,100 miles away lies Boulder, Colorado. For years, Colorado has been the country's benchmark of health, the state with the lowest obesity rates in the United States. And according to a 2011 Gallup and

Healthways survey,[2] out of 190 metropolitan areas studied, Boulder was the least obese in the country, with an adult obesity rate of only 12.1 percent. Here, rates of lifestyle-related illnesses and conditions such as heart attack, diabetes, and high blood pressure trail those of pretty much every other area of the country. It's not a perfect picture, but compared to the rest of the nation, it is just about as good as it gets.

From the standpoint of obesity and health, Holmes County and Boulder have few things in common, other than appearing in many of the same news reports because they lie on opposite ends of the obesity spectrum. In each story, there's the same question: What are we doing right in Boulder that we are doing wrong in Holmes County?

As it turns out, the answer could very well lie in disparities in areas other than just weight. A closer look at the differences between the two reveals that the residents of Boulder enjoy easy access to taxpayer-supported trails and other activities. The area boasts an unusually high rate of educational attainment when compared to the rest of the country, and the populace tends to be more affluent. Meanwhile, many things that are true of Boulder are completely opposite in Holmes County. Here, residents' environment has traditionally offered relatively few tax-supported health amenities like trails and parks, the poverty rate is high, and rates of education are relatively low.

These advantages and disadvantages may not immediately to mind when we think about the country's weight problem. And yet the fact that they are intertwined so tightly with obesity across the nation means something is going on—a collection of broader, population-wide factors that set the stage for healthy or unhealthy weight.

These factors are government policies. In many ways, the policies wrap together many things we have already discussed, including the social, physical, and economic variables that play a part in weight.

Perhaps as you read this, you will find yourself evaluating the area of the country in which you live. Chances are, you live in a county whose weight issues fall somewhere between the extremes of Holmes County and Boulder. And while the weight situation in your area may not be as extreme as it is in either of these places, you can bet that the government policies where you live do affect how easy or difficult it is for inhabitants like you to achieve and maintain a healthy weight.

But how do these broad, overarching policies influence your weight? And what can you do to push for change in a realm that may seem largely out of your control? We will address these questions in this chapter—and you may be surprised to find out how much power you wield.

In other words, take heart; as with the other issues we have discussed, there are ways you can beat your ZIP code.

The Real Effect Government Policies Have on Our Weight

Looking at the Circles of Influence model (page 10) we introduced at the beginning of this book, you will notice we are getting pretty close to the outermost area of the graph. This means it takes a great deal of personal influence to change the policies that dictate the rules, regulations, and norms of the society in which we live—at least when we are acting on our own.

Yet while most of us have relatively little direct influence on the political process from day to day, the influence of government policies on our weight and behaviors is important. The policies affect everything we do, though not necessarily as directly as what happens in our homes, social circles, and workplaces influences our diets, physical activities, and other factors that show up on our waistlines. But indirectly, the policy decisions made by your local, state, and federal governments determine a great many things—how expensive healthy food is, how cheap junk food is, how many green spaces and walkable areas there are in your community. So while you may, like most people, only deal directly with the political process once a year on election day, the results of this process exert a constant pressure on many areas of your daily life, such as your physical environment and your food environment.

Because this pressure is so pervasive, it can almost be thought of as a hidden influence; we don't see it because it is all around us, affecting our day-to-day lives. And in a society in which messages about weight have been tied so tightly to personal responsibility, the policies that shape our environments can be easily missed. This is an issue that Walter and his colleagues, along with Yale University's Kelly Brownell, PhD, explored in a

Why Do We Rank Where We Do in Weight?

Below we have reproduced a chart from a 2011 paper in the journal *Lancet*.[3] Basically, this chart shows obesity prevalence rates in various countries. Take a look at where the United States appears on this

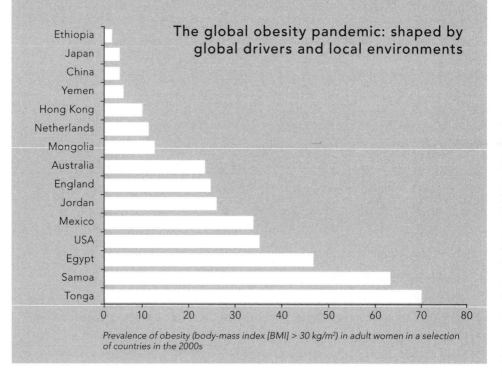

The global obesity pandemic: shaped by global drivers and local environments

Prevalence of obesity (body-mass index [BMI] > 30 kg/m²) in adult women in a selection of countries in the 2000s

report published in the journal *Health Affairs*. The spirit of what they found is well encapsulated in this excerpt from the report:

> The concept of personal responsibility has been central to social, legal, and political approaches to obesity. It evokes language of blame, weakness, and vice and is a leading basis for inadequate government efforts,

chart. For a superpower, not so super. This less-than-admirable ranking may not surprise you, though, if you are familiar with statistics from the Centers for Disease Control and Prevention showing that more than two-thirds of all American adults are either overweight or obese.

But look at where Japan is. It's true: People living in the United States are roughly six times as likely to be heavier than their ideal weight than those living in Japan, despite comparable per capita income levels in the two countries. And now look at where the Netherlands lies in this ranking.

Is there something special about the Japanese and the Dutch that allows them to dodge the weight troubles that we Americans live with? It's not genetics; many Americans can trace their heritage back to these very countries or to other nations that do not have these problems. And to blame it on individual responsibility would suggest that, on the individual level, most every Japanese or Dutch person is somehow more responsible or disciplined than most every American when it comes to decisions that affect their weight. The reason this sounds ridiculous is because it is. Clearly this is not what is happening.

So what are we left with in terms of explanations? In previous chapters, we discussed social and cultural norms specific to the places we live—how often we tend to eat, the types of foods and beverages we regularly enjoy, and even how much of these foods we put on our plate for each meal. But government policies also exert influence over each of these other factors— and the hand they play in the weight problem our country faces cannot be discounted.

given the importance of environmental conditions in explaining high rates of obesity.[4]

In other words, we, as a society, tend to minimize the role that our social and physical environments play in our weight. We instead place the blame on the individual—an approach that, unfortunately, has taken much of the burden off the government with regard to improving school nutrition, curtailing unhealthy industry marketing practices, and even changing (for the better!) the way that our society views healthy eating.

Of course, it is one thing to be aware of this effect; it is something else entirely to exert your influence outward and do something about it. Over the next few pages, we will be guiding you toward ways, both large and small, that you can influence the political landscape in terms of your weight.

What Is "Policy" Anyway?

When you hear the word *politics*, what comes to mind? Most of us picture a congressional chamber, politicians delivering talking points on twenty-four-hour news channels, or the highly publicized rhetoric that typifies the way our government is seen to do its business.

The truth is that while people usually think of policy as a remote issue that involves people in Washington, DC, it actually occurs at every level, from family policy up to global policy. In its purest form, policy is nothing more than the application of rules and guidelines that shape the framework of how we live day to day.

Some government policies are aimed specifically at the issues surrounding obesity; others are not, but they can still have a surprising effect on weight. Take, for example, a ban on single-serving plastic water bottles that went into effect in Concord, Massachusetts, in early 2013. The policy was enacted with the best of intentions; proponents had pushed for years to cut out the use of the single-serving bottles, which they rightfully maintained tend to end up in landfills and generate an inordinate amount of waste. Yet oddly the ban had no effect on soda or juice sold in similar-size bottles. So it takes little creativity to guess what consumers decided to reach for next in the name of convenience. This ban represents just one example of how well-meaning policies—even those that carry real benefits from one point of view—can have a detrimental effect on the obesogenic nature of our environment.

Other examples have far more powerful effects. In addition to providing more than three-quarters of a trillion dollars for food stamps and other nutrition programs (we'll address this ahead), the US farm bill provides billions of taxpayer dollars' worth of assistance to various aspects of commercial food production each year. A large proportion of this support goes to research on commodity crops and educational programs for farmers to produce more of these crops, as well as subsidies and tax measures to encourage the production of corn. Yet there are no such subsidies for fruits and vegetables. This means that there are no incentives for farmers to produce the very foods that Americans would do better to consume more often! And that's not all. While this assistance helps prop up a limited number of jobs, it also subsidizes the production of corn syrup, one of the cheapest and most ubiquitous sweeteners in soda and junk food. As you will see, this isn't the only way that the seemingly good intentions of this bill lead to problems that could end up affecting Americans' weight.

It is important to remember that government policies can appear on all levels and in different forms. The effect they have on your waistline, then, depends very much on your ability to recognize them and act accordingly to either take advantage of them or, when possible, notice and avoid any detrimental effects they may have.

Which brings us back to what you can do. Once you understand what policies are and how they work, you may be able to enact some policies of your own within your immediate environment. This understanding may even help you encourage change within your community and locality to the benefit of all who live there. This is the very essence of grassroots

Policy in (In)Action: The Case of SNAP

A disappointing example of the effects of policy on weight can be found in a program set up ostensibly to help one of the most vulnerable segments of our population. The program is the Supplemental Nutrition Assistance Program, or SNAP (formally the food stamp program).

Researchers have been mulling the relationship between poverty and obesity for years. As a result, the relationship between weight and economic status has become one of the most heavily studied areas in obesity research to date, and there is strong evidence that being in a lower socioeconomic bracket is linked to risk of unhealthy weight. In other words, the poor are not only vulnerable economically but also at great risk of unhealthy weight.

Enter SNAP. One in seven Americans relies on the extra money provided by SNAP to make ends meet. However, aside from prohibitions on certain items, such as tobacco and alcohol, currently no guidelines dictate the nutritional value of the food that is purchased.

The thing is, an analysis out of the Harvard University School of Public Health, published in the *American Journal of Clinical Nutrition* and based on national survey data, found that SNAP participants were more likely to be obese or to have the metabolic warning signs of diabetes than others in the general population with similar incomes.[5] Naturally, given that the program costs US taxpayers upward of $75 billion each year and that it makes up about 80 percent of the entire US farm bill, researchers wanted to find out how much SNAP money was going to healthful, nutritious fare and how much went to junk food.

In a 2010 paper published in *The American Journal of Public Health*,[6] researchers Jonathan Shenkin, DDS, MPH, of Boston University and Michael Jacobson, PhD, of the Center for Science in the Public Interest

change. Many past efforts that have started with relatively humble local beginnings have led to important policy changes. Reductions of and bans on trans fats in food, smoke-free laws in restaurants and public places—these are just a couple of examples of local initiatives that have highlighted this question. Dr. Jacobson, using data he had gathered in that year at one major supermarket chain, found that soda accounted for more than 6 percent of the grocery bills of those using food stamps. "Thus," he extrapolated, "if food-stamp expenditures in fiscal year 2011 are about $69 billion, then almost $4 billion will be spent on carbonated soft drinks." The authors further noted that "[t]his sum could be considered a direct subsidy to the soft drink and supermarket industries."

Drs. Shenkin and Jacobson are not alone in their conclusion. Many others feel the evidence shows the SNAP program is so dominated by special interests from within the food industry that there is an impossibly strong current against healthy changes that would set us on a course to solving the country's weight woes. Making matters worse, many of the nation's urban and rural poor live in areas where healthy options are either too expensive or not readily accessible.

If we had only these observations to guide us, it would be fairly easy to guess how this combination of factors might affect the health of those who depend on the SNAP program. But we may not have to resort to guessing; Walter and his colleagues have conducted research on this very issue. A study led by Cindy Leung, DSc, and published in the *American Journal of Clinical Nutrition*[7] found that few adults receiving SNAP adhered to a healthy diet. In fact, on average they consumed almost three servings of sugar-sweetened beverages per day, and a few even consumed five to six servings per day. Conversely, very few of these adults ate recommended amounts of healthy whole grains, vegetables, fruit, fish, nuts, and legumes. This suggests that SNAP money is often spent on cheap sources of calories rather than on wholesome foods.

Policies could make important differences, such as requiring stores that redeem food stamps to offer healthy options. Thus far, the USDA, which administers SNAP and is strongly influenced by major food industries, has refused requests by cities or states to improve the nutritional quality of the program. It is an unfortunate example of policy working in favor of profits for specific industries and against efforts to control the obesity epidemic.

spread more widely, providing an enormous benefit to public health.

Helping to make the changes that affect your community, your locality, or even the country as a whole is a lofty goal. But small steps to call for positive change, if taken by a large number of people, can sometimes lead

Do Healthy Policies Violate Your Civil Rights?

Recently, the common refrain of those who oppose certain government policies promoting healthy food options and discouraging unhealthy choices has been that such policies infringe on freedom of choice. In the most extreme examples of these arguments, some have maintained that the policies go so far as to violate civil rights.

One proposed policy that garnered a great deal of attention was former New York City mayor Michael Bloomberg's suggestion that restaurants and other establishments be prevented from offering sugary drinks, such as soda, in serving sizes larger than sixteen ounces. The ban would not prevent a consumer from ordering a second beverage of the same size or from buying large bottles of soda from the grocery store; in essence, it would only limit the size of each serving you would get at a restaurant or a movie theater.

In a May 2012 interview with ABC News's Diane Sawyer, Bloomberg defended the policy, citing that in New York City alone, obesity has a major impact on the well-being of residents, as well as the city's economy.

"Obesity deaths are at five thousand and skyrocketing," Bloomberg told Sawyer. "Obesity will kill more people than smoking in the next couple of years."

But on the day the policy was scheduled to go into effect, a New York Supreme Court judge dismissed the ban—a decision Bloomberg quickly said he planned to appeal.

According to many estimates, calories from soda and other sugary beverages are the top source of calories in the American diet. So the policy would at least seem well tailored to the problem. Yet the argument has always been that this policy, as well as others that encourage consumers to think twice before making unhealthy decisions, interferes with freedom of choice.

The first thing that we, as a society, must realize about such arguments—as well as "nanny state" and "big brother" rhetoric—is that many of these messages are actively promoted by those who have vested economic interests. These interests may come in the form of companies that sell the products in question or from lobbying groups supported by these industries.

The second thing is that these policies—and the relatively minor inconvenience that they pose to some—tend to have a significant positive impact for society as a whole in the long term. As an example, when was the last time you went out to eat at a restaurant and someone at the next table lit up a cigarette? Or boarded a flight to discover you were seated next to the smoking section? Smoke-free laws are often, and rightfully, cited as a triumph of public health in cutting back deaths linked to lung cancer from smoking. These policies no doubt inconvenienced a certain segment of the population when they were enacted. Yet health statistics show that we, as a society, are better off for it, both in health and economic terms.

As Walter, Kelly Brownell, and their colleagues pointed out in their 2010 *Health Affairs* paper:

> Public health approaches, particularly those involving government action, are sometimes caricatured as forcing people to behave in certain ways. In fact, though, the public health community has long understood the need for programs that blend a focus on individual choices and collective responsibility. Contemporary advances have resulted from such interventions as improved sanitation, control of infectious diseases,

better nutrition, and reduced smoking.

In short, all of us are entitled to our own opinions about the line between our rights and government regulation. But it is worth noting that a sixteen- or eighteen-year-old who has developed diabetes due to excessive consumption of soda—having been subjected to thousands of ads associating soda with happiness, social connectedness, good looks, and popular sports events—has also lost a huge amount of freedom of choice. The idea that we all might have to walk to the counter for a second serving of soda seems rather trivial compared to loss of choice for that child.

And it is not just that child who will be affected. When he or she develops renal failure and needs dialysis, we as taxpayers all pick up the tab, whether the person had private, public, or no insurance. And at every level of government, health care costs—to a large extent influenced by our lifestyle choices—are displacing budgets for education, parks, research, the arts, and other elements that make our society vibrant and strong.

These connections may be less direct than the effects of someone smoking in a seat next to us, but nevertheless, our decisions do have profound effects beyond own lives; hence the need to consider and debate the balancing of individual choice and societal impacts.

to real results—and your influence may be just what some of these efforts need to become reality.

How You Can Influence Policy

So far we have highlighted how overarching policies can affect your health-related behaviors. This is one side of the coin. But you may be wondering how you can go about using your own influence to affect policy.

The good news is that, while influencing matters on this level may not be as simple as influencing change in your own behaviors or among those in your close social circles, you can make it happen. Below we will go through the various levels at which you can encourage healthy policies.

Starting at Home:
Your Household Food "Policies"

While we have talked quite a bit in this chapter about the effect of government policies, the policies you put into place in your home environment are perhaps even more important in enforcing the behaviors that can keep your own weight, as well as the weight of those who live in your household, under control.

What form might these policies take? In your home, you might be able to take a huge step in the right direction by "banning" full-sugar sodas. If your family is like most in the United States, this step alone would cut out a major source of dietary sugar. If this seems like too drastic an adjustment, you might decide instead to take a page from New York City and limit the size of sodas and other sugary beverages within your home. Consider it for a second. You could get smaller glasses designated to be used only for soda. The end result would be more refills—a conscious choice that gives you a chance to pause and think about what you are doing, as well as how much you actually want that second serving of soda. It seems almost too simple, yet studies have shown[8,9] how this little bit of mindfulness can cut down on the overall consumption of calories. So a small adjustment like this might make sense.

Other policies may involve limiting the areas of the home where meals can be enjoyed. A strict "no food on the couch" policy may be a bit of a sore spot with your family at first. But in the long run, instituting such a policy could drastically cut down the snacking calories consumed within your household, thus easily eliminating one of the most common barriers to a healthier weight. Yet another option might be to limit TV watching, which is consistently associated with weight gain and diabetes.

Is instituting a policy necessary for these changes? It might not hurt. Having a clear policy can help avoid constantly revisiting an issue, especially when it is a negotiated policy agreed upon by all involved. The trick with these household policies is, in many ways, the same as what is seen in more overarching policies—small steps, properly enforced, can lead to positive change. Often the worst thing you can do within your home is create a policy that is overly restrictive or burdensome. Bear this in mind when you are laying down the law for yourself or for those you love.

Getting a Good Start for the Kids: School Policies

Much policy research has focused on institutional measures to address widespread weight problems—and as one of the more recognizable institutions in our society, the school is naturally an area where these problems are being addressed.

The most scrutinized element of the school equation is the issue of the food and drinks available to children in the school setting. So it should come as little surprise that many of the efforts to change school policy have focused on what children are eating and drinking while at school.

One particularly notable policy success has been elimination of soda from schools. Harvard School of Public Health's Steve Gortmaker, PhD, has shown that this policy in Boston schools resulted in a 17 percent reduction in total soda consumption by children.[10] And while the policy was only technically in effect in the schools, it also highlighted the need to address consumption at home for further progress.

Also worth noting is that this success in Boston was largely due to the committed activity of a small number of parents and resulted in a national compact, organized by the Clinton Foundation, to maintain high standards for beverages served in schools.

So if you happen to be a parent of a school-age child, does this mean that you have to barge into your child's school cafeteria, demanding change? Fortunately, the answer to this question is no (and, as an aside, we would further advise against taking such action in the interest of sparing your child the mortifying experience). Rather, start by attending a local school board meeting, as Malissa has done in the past. She quickly found the incredible impact that a thoughtful, fact-based presentation can have in this type of setting. The simple point to bear in mind is that, when children's health is at stake, policy makers at this level will often listen to community concerns.

Making a Difference in Community Policies

Speaking of communities, you can use your influence to help encourage weight-friendly policies through many different venues. Think about the groups to which you may belong—a community association, a local chapter of a national organization, a church, a mosque, or a synagogue. These are all potential backdrops for healthy efforts.

Faith-based settings, in particular, may be great venues to influence others to get behind a program to achieve healthy weight through policies that encourage healthier behaviors. One of the latest studies illustrating this principle showed up in the journal *Preventing Chronic Disease*.[11] This study showed that advocacy of weight loss messages in a rural, African

American church led to significant average weight loss among members of the congregation.

The inroad to change usually involves approaching the governing bodies of the groups and presenting to them the idea of new, healthy

The Environmental Impact of Our Food Choices

In this book, we focus on social and environmental factors that influence our weight and well-being. Today many people are also concerned about the effects of our behaviors on the health of our environment.

This is for good reason. Human health is ultimately dependent on the quality of the air we breathe, the water we drink, and productivity of our land and seas. Many of these resources are under stress and not sustainable for future generations unless current trends are changed.

Fortunately most of the same dietary and activity patterns that promote an optimal weight and overall well-being also contribute to the health of our environment. Our choices of protein sources provide a good example. High consumption of beef, which contributes to heart disease, diabetes, and weight gain,

also produces approximately five to ten times the amount of carbon dioxide and other greenhouse gases per calorie compared to beans, lentils, or poultry. And we don't need to be strict vegetarians to make a big difference; replacing red meat with chicken reduces greenhouse gas production by about 75 percent.[12] Similar differences are seen for water and energy requirements.

On the activity side, the differences are even larger. Walking, riding a bike, or taking public transportation compared to driving a car has major health benefits and also massively reduces energy consumption and greenhouse gas production. Walter has calculated that he gets more than one thousand miles per gallon of olive oil when he rides his bike to work!

policies within the organization. Once you have an idea for a policy change, see if you can get others on board. Remember, when it comes to getting a good idea to flourish, there is strength in numbers!

Taking Steps to Improve Local Policies

Former US Speaker of the House Tip O'Neill is widely credited with coining the phrase "All politics is local." Granted, he probably didn't have public health specifically in mind when he said this. But the phrase rings true for weight-healthy policies as well—particularly considering that such

We're All in This Together

If there is a reason why the vast majority of weight loss books do not delve into policy in the way we have throughout this chapter, it may be that, traditionally, weight has largely been considered an individual issue. We spend a great deal of time looking in the mirror at ourselves and our midsections. We spend less time holding this mirror up to the rest of the society in which we live.

We have looked at the impacts of excess weight on the health of others in our immediate vicinity, as well as the way our choices can impact our environment. But what about the ways that it can affect our prosperity as a society and as a nation?

Estimating the costs of obesity to society is tricky business. What we do know is that, economically speaking, the consequences of the combined excess weight of our country is nothing short of disastrous. Some estimates have pegged the economic cost to society at $147 billion—with a hefty portion of this tab picked up by the taxpayer-supported programs policies often become stuck in governmental gridlock at the national level.

Indeed, you have probably read in the past the news stories about local government policies aimed at curbing weight problems. Many of these have been introduced in our largest cities, including the proposed soda-size initiative in New York City as well as that same government's work to put calorie counts on restaurant menus, among other efforts. And New York City is already beginning to reap the rewards of these actions, it would seem; recent data show rates of obesity within the city have declined in the last several years after many years of steady increases.

Research has also shown that sensible policies, implemented locally,

Medicare and Medicaid.[13] Even in the shadow of these sobering estimates, other researchers have suggested that the total bill is far worse. For example, John Cawley, PhD, of Cornell University and Chad Meyerhoefer, PhD, of Lehigh University have estimated that in 2005 the United States collectively spent $190 billion on obesity.[14] Their estimate, unlike some in the past, looked at both the direct costs of obesity—such as surgery, medications, and hospital costs—and the indirect costs—lost work, lower wages, and insurance costs.

No matter how we measure it, these are mind-boggling numbers. We also need to realize that these dollars are coming from somewhere. And given the nature of insurance and the other ways we, as a society, pool risks, it soon becomes clear that we are all footing the bill.

Should we view this realization as the ultimate societal guilt trip the next time we see the numbers spin by as we step on the scale? Of course not—that's really not what this chapter is all about. Rather, we hope that you view this connection to society's pocketbook as the ultimate incentive for widespread change. The truth is that we are all in this together. And while we may feel that it is difficult to affect the big picture, all of our individual changes, taken together, can go a very long way in influencing the costs that we all bear.

can have a substantial positive impact. At least one such analysis, conducted in the United Kingdom by Dr. Charlie Foster and colleagues and published in the journal *Obesity Reviews*, suggests means by which local governments can reduce the obesogenic quotient of communities, leading to healthier lifestyles for the population at large.[15] In another example, a paper by Yale researchers Jennifer Harris, PhD, and Samantha Graff, JD, explored policy options for municipalities seeking ways to limit harmful

Dan's Story:

GETTING TO KNOW THE GREEN CARTS

In 2010 my wife and I made the transition from the suburbs of Boston to Manhattan. We had a lot of things on our mind—selling a recently purchased condo, hunting for an apartment for rent on short notice. But one of the most unanticipated changes to our lifestyle was in the way this move would affect the way we got our food.

Gone were the days of the two-mile weekend drive to the nearest supermarket; we had sold our car in anticipation of the parking nightmare that otherwise awaited us. The other adjustment—no more pantry. Add to this the fact that our apartment refrigerator was roughly one-quarter the size of the spacious icebox we used to enjoy. So storing an entire week's worth of fresh food was pretty much out of the question.

food marketing at the community level—a level at which individual advocacy may make a bigger difference than you'd think.[16]

So how can you get involved in this larger process of government policy making? The most important part of promoting a good idea for policies on the local level is for you to be present within your local government. Perhaps the ideas you would like to push forward resemble the examples we have already provided, such as forming bicycle and pedestrian committees to

For our first few months in the city, the Green Carts were a godsend. These carts, we learned, were set up through a New York City permit-issuing program back in 2008. The new permits, one thousand in all, were granted to street vendors with the understanding that they would sell only raw fruits and vegetables. They would be strategically placed throughout the city to deal with what the city solons viewed as a social problem—the lack of easily accessible fresh produce throughout the city's concrete jungle landscape.

Augmenting the city's efforts were groups such as Accion USA and the Laurie M. Tisch Illumination Fund, which provided low-interest loans and grants for business consulting to the entrepreneurs who ran the Green Carts. In many ways, it is a textbook model of how local government policies, bolstered by nongovernmental investments, can lead to a meaningful step toward improving the health of the population as a whole.

For us, of course, the carts meant fresh nectarines and asparagus instead of the limited corner store fare—as well as a convenient way to avoid falling into an unhealthy and obesogenic food trap.

develop and improve standards for streets and facilities to encourage more physical activity in your community. Or maybe it's another idea altogether. Don't be afraid to do what you need to do to garner support for your good idea among others, or to pitch in with others in your community toward a plan for positive change. A little bit of grassroots organization can go a long way, and it is a fantastic testing ground for your influence.

Influencing the Big Picture

As we have mentioned, making changes on the federal level is a lofty goal, and it can turn out to be frustrating and fruitless if you try to do it on your own. Fortunately you can lend your influence to what is happening nationally in other ways.

Your first step may be to research various groups already pushing for the changes you would like to see in your community and beyond. While a number of groups share weight-related goals, a quick and easy way to get started is to contact your local American Heart Association chapter at www.myamericanheart.org and ask to be connected with the advocacy staff member. Once you have gotten in touch, you can sign up to be on a mailing list for obesity and/or childhood obesity, and you can also receive prewritten letters on these issues to e-mail directly to your congressional representatives and senators. Another option is to write your own e-mails and letters to your representative asking them to support measures that would improve public health in terms of obesity and weight. Additionally, you may be able to advocate through your city and state government offices.

Thinfluence Action Plan: Applying Your Influence to Policy

Depending on your situation, you may never have the opportunity—or, frankly, the desire—to carry your influence into the realm of policy change. That's fine! If this describes your situation, the important take-home message for you is to recognize the influence that various policies have on the other areas of your life—whether at your workplace, at the grocery store, or in your family's food budget—and to come up with the best strategies possible to work with (or around) this backdrop. Understanding the situation you are dealing with is an important step in getting that extra leverage to achieve your weight goals.

If, however, you are interested in joining the cause to advocate for a less obesogenic environment where you and your family live, there are ways to get on board. Go in with your eyes open, knowing that it will take some effort, but it could be a very rewarding endeavor indeed!

ANALYZE

1. How would you rate the current policies within your community regarding public health?

    A. Few, if any, policies or initiatives are in place in my community to deal with issues that affect health and weight, such as the availability of healthful foods. There is also little to suggest that past initiatives have had an effect (increased availability of parks and green spaces, efforts to encourage healthier eating, etc.).

    B. Some policies appear to be in place in my community to deal with important public health issues like obesity and poor lifestyle habits. At least occasionally I see an initiative encouraging healthy behaviors that is supported by my local government, and there is some evidence that past initiatives have led to changes in the community, such as new or refurbished green spaces and exercise areas.

    C. It is very clear to me that my local government holds healthy lifestyles as a high priority. Multiple government-backed initiatives in the past have led to policy changes within my community, and the programs that are put into place usually have a great deal of public support.

2. **Think about the grassroots efforts within your community. What best describes the situation in the community where you live?**

    A. Few if any groups appear to be active within my community when it comes to health issues. While there may be a number of community groups—churches and local chapters of service organizations, for example—they do not seem to confront important health issues that deal with the weight of those living in the area.

    B. While no community groups are taking the lead in pushing for policies and initiatives that would improve health and weight on the whole, I do notice the occasional effort to encourage healthy lifestyles.

    C. Numerous groups in my community are pushing for policies that encourage positive lifestyle changes, perhaps even those that specifically deal with weight issues. Many of these groups work together to advance their healthy agendas, and there is wide community "buy-in" for these efforts.

3. **Now think about your own involvement in community efforts to change policies that affect health. What best describes your approach?**

    A. While encouraging such policies may be important to me, I have not taken an active role within my community to push for such changes. Also, I am currently not a part of any groups within the community that I feel might advocate for health- and weight-related policies where I live.

    B. I belong to some groups—such as religious groups or community service organizations—that might consider pushing for policies that would encourage healthy lifestyles. Depending on the form these efforts took, I would consider getting involved.

C. I am actively involved in one or more groups that advocate for policies that improve the health- and lifestyle-related behaviors of those living in my community.

ACT

When you look at your answers to these questions, what do you see?

◊ **Mostly As:** It appears that you live in a community in which the local government and other entities are not currently engaged in any real health-promoting initiatives. However, as long as factors in your community contribute to unhealthy weight behaviors, there is a real need for change. Can you be the source of this change? The only way to find out is to get involved. Start asking local groups about their involvement in health-related efforts. Think about forming a neighborhood group to approach your local government. Given that the health of your community is at stake, it is most certainly worth the effort.

◊ **Mostly Bs:** The fact that some groups are already making inroads to your community's weight issues is a plus. See what you can do to get involved—whether this involves joining a neighborhood group, being more active in your church's efforts to encourage healthy behaviors, or bringing up issues of weight and health at PTA meetings or other gatherings. You may find that your contributions to existing efforts can translate into real change, both for yourself and for your community.

◊ **Mostly Cs:** It sounds like your community is a rare standout with policies that encourage weight-friendly lifestyle habits. Make sure that you are involved in these efforts, and don't be afraid to speak up and share your ideas and opinions. Better yet, see if you can use your influence to get your friends and family involved in these efforts as well.

No matter what the situation is in your community, anyone can take steps to push for healthier policies. Here are a few ideas to get you started:

◊ Reach out to your community reporters. Local media coverage can go a long way in terms of promoting ideas for your community to help influence others toward a healthier weight.

◊ Take advantage of the motivation to lose weight in your church group to start some activities in conjunction with the aforementioned local health organizations.

◊ Be a positive example within your community! As in other areas of your life, there is no substitute for showing those around you the changes that are possible through healthier choices.

INFLUENCE

More than any other Circle of Influence we have discussed in this book, the circle that ensconces policy has the potential to change weight-related behaviors on a large scale. But it is also the one for which sowing the seeds of change can be most challenging. If you decide to take on this challenge, the most important arrows in your quiver will be the potential incentives you can use to influence others to support your efforts. Here are some of the possible outcomes that can help in this regard:

◊ Greater health awareness and consciousness within your community and social groups, leading to a healthier lifestyle and a better weight

◊ Improved social ties and support for healthful activities

◊ An overall healthier community and a greater awareness of healthy measures in other community institutions. You might even want to consider some of the more inspiring examples that we discussed in this chapter—improved food and beverages in schools, for example, or the New York City Green Cart initiative. These programs are largely the result of grassroots efforts. What are your best ideas?

Once again, it is important to bear in mind that policy can be at any level: personal, family, neighborhood, city, state, national, even global. Often city policies can be more easily achieved because pushback from powerful special interest groups may be less, but this is harder at state and national levels. Still, local action can become national, as we have seen for trans fat bans in restaurants, smoking bans in restaurants and work sites, and other efforts that started in some cities, then became statewide, and now cover large parts of the country.

How far can your influence extend within your household, your community, and your country as far as policies are concerned? There is only one way to find out: Get involved!

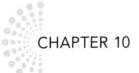

CHAPTER 10

Thinfluence: Putting It All Together

Throughout this book, we have discussed a wide range of strategies for using various levels of influence to bring about changes that encourage healthier weight. And while each of these strategies alone has the potential to help you change your waistline and your health for the better, the effects will likely be even more profound and lasting when the strategies are combined.

With this in mind, imagine what would happen in a place where all of these levels of influence were addressed at once. You might envision a community in which families and other social networks have realized their full potential as conduits of healthy behaviors and lifestyle habits. Individual efforts would be supported by a combination of measures designed to improve the physical environment and the food environment. Corporate institutions, government agencies, and not-for-profit organizations would work hand in hand to implement policies to improve health, and all who were involved would reap the benefits.

In short, you might envision a scenario much like the one created by a recent pilot program in Bell County, Kentucky, to help improve the health of its inhabitants.

Bell County, which sits at Kentucky's borders with Virginia and Tennessee, is home to just under thirty thousand people. It is a county like so many in the United States, where more than one in three adults are obese. Weight-linked health problems are high here as well; 12.4 percent of adults have type 2 diabetes, compared to the state rate of 9.9 percent.

Given Kentucky's status as one of the states with the highest rates of obesity in the nation, it is no surprise that many of these residents struggle with an unhealthy weight and the assortment of health problems that often accompany it. Wilhelmina, who grew up in this tight-knit community and lives there to this day, was just one such resident.

Prior to the program, Wilhelmina says, her weight hovered around three hundred pounds. She knew there was a problem, but her efforts to fix it and get to a healthier weight invariably failed—a pattern that over the years had taken a big toll on her emotionally and psychologically.

"I have been overweight all my life," Wilhelmina, a sixty-one-year-old grandmother, told us. "I've tried different things with doctors with programs and everything. They didn't seem to stick no matter how hard I tried."

Occasionally her desire to improve her weight and health put her health at risk. "I've even taken diet pills in my life," she confided. "One of my diet pills I was taking did work a lot, but then it was taken off market because they found out it was bad for people. It was just a yo-yo way of life, and sometimes I'd go home and sit down and cry. I would try to do everything I possibly could do, then my doctor tells me I'm not doing it or I'm not trying."

So when she heard about a new pilot health program coming to Bell County, she looked forward to finding out more. "I guess you could say I was hoping this would be something that would really help me this time."

The program was Team Up 4 Health, and one of the minds behind its development is Daniel Zoughbie, who in 2005 founded the not-for-profit organization known today as Microclinic International (MCI). Dedicated to the memory of Zoughbie's grandmother who died of diabetes, MCI was based on a simple yet profound idea: that healthy lifestyle-related behaviors could be contagious, spreading from person to person through social networks and communities.

Before coming to Bell County, MCI had already compiled an impressive batting average in other communities around the globe. At the heart of each previous effort was a strategy that sought not to supplant the existing infrastructure of the community, but rather to use this infrastructure to its fullest as a conduit for healthy behaviors.

Wilhelmina was one of 265 participants in the Team Up 4 Health pilot program in Bell County. And as her experience showed, the program used approaches that addressed several layers of the Circles of Influence graph (page 10) that we have been discussing throughout this book.

The program made inroads into changes on the policy level by teaming up with the Bell County Health Department, which worked with Team Up 4 Health to manage the day-to-day program. MCI also got other organizations on board that had a vested interest in the health of the community. On the academic side was a team led by Eric Ding, ScD, of MCI from Harvard University School of Public Health. From the corporate side was the health insurance company Humana, which sponsored the pilot phase of the program.

To coach program participants in improving their food environments, the organizers assembled larger groups for counseling and education on such topics as nutrition and healthy food selection. The program also included group trips to the grocery store, where participants would get together and learn how to build a healthier cart. "We had a different thing each week," Wilhelmina says. "We'd have a class on reading labels. We had a nutritionist come in, and she talked to us about different things. We were shown how much sugar was in this, how much sugar was in that. They showed you how to cook low-calorie meals, and you would get to sample it to see if you liked it or not." Further improving the food environment throughout Bell County, the program placed a new emphasis on community gardening, teaching participants how to grow and harvest their own produce.

As for improving the physical environment, she says the Health Department installed two new sets of exercise equipment in the county. She sees this equipment being used regularly by program participants and their families, a sign that this simple change to the physical environment turned out to be contagious.

But the most important ingredient for change in the program turned out to be the way it exploited the social environment—the family and friendship networks of the participants. The true aim of the research side of the program, in fact, was to see what would happen if participants were allowed to make the most of the strong social support networks that already existed in the county. To do this, half of the participants in the program were instructed to bring in a few of their close family members and friends whom they felt would be supportive of their efforts. For Wilhelmina, this meant taking her brother along for the ride.

The two- to six-member "microgroups" that resulted from this strategy became the basic building blocks of this part of the program. Doctors, nutritionists, and other health professionals would begin by asking the groups what their goals were—goals for the week ahead, goals for the long term. These health professionals then provided guidance on exercise and nutrition that could help participants achieve these goals. But the true support came from the fact that the participants in the microgroups had known each other for decades and had shared their lives with one another. So when they decided to get healthier, they were able to motivate and support each other in their efforts. These microgroups were further supported by the Bell County community as a whole.

"It was always support, support, support," Wilhelmina says. "There never was one negative thing said. That meant a lot, because I had experienced a lot of negativity over the years. Instead they say, 'Wilhelmina, you're looking good. You're looking better than I seen you look in a long time.'"

So what changes did the program bring about? Wilhelmina's eleven-year-old granddaughter, who was part of her microgroup, stopped drinking sugary soda, opting instead for milk and water. Like her grandmother, she started trying new foods.

Indeed, a look back at the data collected after the first phase of the pilot program revealed that while most everyone who participated in the program benefited, those who were allowed to form their own tightly knit microgroups appeared to enjoy the most noticeable benefits. Among these participants, more than 97 percent improved in at least one of four areas (reduced body mass index, sustained weight loss, decreased symptoms of diabetes, and reduced blood pressure) by the end of the first year. On average, these participants lost six and a half pounds. They were several times more likely to engage in various forms of physical activity. More than half reported increasing their consumption of healthy nuts and legumes.

And for Wilhelmina, the results were obvious.

"I have lost right now close to sixty pounds and kept it off," she says. "It could be a little bit more than that for all I know. The thing is, I didn't really go into this program as a weight loss program. I went into it to learn how to get healthy. . . . To me, the weight loss is like dessert."

These are just the kinds of changes, those behind the program say, that drive home the idea that introducing healthy changes within social networks and communities can be powerful in turning the tide of obesity and chronic lifestyle-related conditions.

"There's this incredibly beautiful human story here," Zoughbie says of those who are reaping the benefits of the program, which is now going into its second phase in Bell County. "Our goal is to support that human story with some really heavy-hitting scientific data that backs up the sort of thing that Wilhelmina is sharing with us."

"There is a lot of data that negative behaviors—like drinking or smoking or overeating—spread through people's social network," says Leila Makarechi, a colleague of Zoughbie's at MCI. "So if diseases are contagious, why can't we reverse things for the better and make health contagious? Engaging not just a single patient or person, but also a social support system is a much more effective way, and frankly a simple way, to have improvements in health outcomes."

Could harnessing the positive effects of encouraging healthier behaviors in small group settings be an effective weapon against the nationwide obesity epidemic? Zoughbie thinks so.

"What we envision is something that could ripple throughout the entire state and perhaps through the entire nation," Zoughbie says. "Someone on our staff suggested that this is a program that could set the nation on fire, so to speak. In our minds, we really see this as something that could save, once brought to scale, millions of lives and billions of dollars. There is no goal more worthy or ambitious, but we believe it's achievable."

Assessing Your Infrastructure

The Bell County story has many interesting facets. But perhaps one of the most interesting features becomes apparent when you consider the combination of various approaches employed by the Team Up 4 Health program. It is easy to see how no one single factor caused this shift in lifestyle for so many people. Rather, it was a blend of many different factors—strong community ties, a supportive local government, and the energy of many individuals—that made this approach a success story.

Throughout this book, we have shared compelling stories about people for whom weight is a serious concern. Many have faced special challenges, while others are beginning their journeys toward a healthier weight. Still others have enjoyed success in their weight loss efforts and are now hoping to pass along what they have learned. The common thread through all of these stories has been the way these individuals have sought to take advantage of the positive influence surrounding their efforts, recognized the negative influences that threaten to hinder them, and even become helpful influences themselves within their families, social networks, and communities.

But the example of Bell County stands out; it demonstrates what can happen when many of the various tumblers fall into place. In this story, the healthy and encouraging infrastructure that rose from a multilevel effort offered participants in this program the best of all worlds, all at once. Those who were fortunate enough to be part of this program were effectively immersed in a healthy new lifestyle.

So as you approach the end of this book, it is a great time to examine your own "infrastructure." How well do the various Circles of Influence in your life match up and work together to help you reach your goals? What is the sum total of all of the positive and negative influences in your life when it comes to controlling your weight? And what, if anything, can you do to bring your surroundings more in line with an environment that will help you achieve your weight goals?

In the remaining pages, we hope to help you shed light on all these aspects of your life, as well as help you go through our Thinfluence Action Plan to determine the best strategies in your toolbox that you can start using today (if you haven't started using them already!).

As we do this, the important thing to remember is that nobody has been dealt a perfect hand. Each of us must address an assortment of challenges and disadvantages to achieve the weight we want. The trick is to recognize the various changes we can make—not only to our own actions, but to the other myriad aspects of our lives we have discussed so far—to more easily achieve our goals.

Where to Start? Determining Which Goal to Tackle First

While we're on the topic of goals, it is time to ask yourself the obvious question: Why did I pick up this book?

In all likelihood you reached for it because of your own desire to lose weight, and, like Wilhelmina, you found that the approaches you've tried in the past have not worked. Perhaps your desire to learn how to better help a loved one lose weight prompted you to pick it up, or maybe you were interested in creating a healthier home environment for your entire family. Whatever the reason, we hope you have found out more about how your influence can extend beyond yourself when it comes to behaviors that encourage a healthy weight. Your goal now—whether it involves changing your own weight, influencing your loved ones or friends to achieve a healthier weight, or becoming an influential force for positive change in your community—may not be the same as when you opened up the first chapter. Whether or not this is the case, you should realize by now that most approaches to achieving a healthier diet and a better weight can work, even while most diet efforts themselves fail. Often the missing ingredient involves leveraging the power of social influence within your various networks and environments to help you achieve your goals—and make your progress last.

So now that you likely have your goal in view, the next step is to decide how best to approach it. The answer in most cases is to start in the Circle of Influence in which you feel there is the most room for positive change. For some people, this may be right at the center of the Circles of Influence, with your inner factors. If this is the case, seeking some specialized counseling or getting some other kind of help for stress or depression on a very personal level may be the best first step you can take. As you consider the dynamics at the center of the Circles of Influence graph (page 10), you may also decide that for you, the first step may be in dealing with the family environment or situations within your work environment.

To be clear, we are not saying you should develop tunnel vision in the steps you take; indeed, that approach would stand in contrast to the entire message of this book. Rather we are advising you to think about your priorities, which are in part a function of how big the impact would be of the various actions you could take. If you decide that starting with your home environment would make the biggest impact for you and your family, working on that area first may well give you the best momentum to use in other areas of your life. Your priorities are also shaped by whom you would like to help. It may be that you are reading this book to find some new ideas and approaches to help a close friend achieve his or her weight goals. If so, the priority may be to make changes within your social circle that will help achieve this goal.

Once you have begun to address the area in which the biggest opportunity exists, you can start to address other areas of your social and/or physical environment to pave the way for real, lasting changes. This means that if you decide your primary area for change is your social circle, you may work on that first—but you might find later that exerting your positive influence toward a healthier neighborhood environment supports this goal as well.

This mode of thinking may also help to identify the areas where you know you will have the greatest impact. If you are a leader in your church, for example, that group may be a good place to garner support for your healthy ideas. Or if you are active in your broader community or local government, this involvement may be the foot in the door that you need to gather support for your healthy ideas and help them to spread. Bear in mind that there is nothing wrong with a challenge. But if a challenge is too great or too ambitious for the time being, there may be other opportunities to make positive changes. Don't hesitate to reach for the low-hanging fruit first; the beauty of Thinfluence is that many areas of your life will present opportunities for positive change.

No matter what area of your life you decide to tackle first, you will be looking for a lasting lifestyle change, so this kind of holistic approach will be key.

When the Going Gets Tough . . .

For most people, getting to a healthier weight and maintaining that weight over the long term is no small feat. This means that roadblocks,

Thinfluence in Review: Your Take-Home Messages

Considering the many suggestions and approaches we have presented in this book, the most important next step for you is to decide which ones work for you and deserve a place in your toolbox.

To help you, here is a road map that recaps some of the most important messages within each of the chapters you have read.

Chapter 1: What Is Thinfluence? Think about where you were when you picked up this book and where you are now. You might even want to make a list of the top five things you have learned from this book and hope to incorporate in your life. Every time you start to forget what you have learned, look at the list.

Chapter 2: Know Thyself. Truly ask yourself if your emotions affect your eating and healthy behaviors. If they do, you might want to prepare an emergency emotional eating kit and develop a list of healthy distractions when your willpower is running low.

Chapter 3: Family Matters. Share what you have learned in this book with your family (bit by bit as you see fit). For additional guidance, make a copy of "What Is a Healthy Diet?" (page 19) for your refrigerator as a reminder.

Chapter 4: Friends and Organizations. Use the collective "we" to become the collective "we are fit and healthy." Lead by example in your circle of friends. And be prepared with strategies that will help you interact healthfully with those whose choices may not be in line with yours.

Chapter 5: Your Workplace and Your Waistline. Evaluate the options for health promotion in your workplace. Find out about nutrition and exercise programs. Does your cafeteria provide

dead ends, and hurdles are not only possible—you are in fact likely to encounter them.

The beauty of what we have seen in the previous chapters, however, is that you likely have many more options at your disposal than you options and information to help you make a smart food choice while at work? Is there a way you could make your work environment more conducive to your weight goals?

Chapter 6: Your Food Environment. This chapter could be called Food Feng Shui. For the uninitiated, this refers to the ancient art of arranging your living environment—except in this case, you are arranging your food environment. Look around your home and take note of changes you can make to improve access to the foods you know are healthy. This is another instance in which a copy of "What Is a Healthy Diet" (page 19) may come in handy. Clear out the cabinets and start fresh. After all, if it's not there, you won't eat it.

Chapter 7: Your Physical Environment. Maximize your opportunities to eat as a family and remember to minimize eating in front of the television. Try to incorporate more exercise into your daily life. Make it part of your commute to and from work if possible.

Chapter 8: Your Media "Diet." Remember that the effect of advertising on our health is more pronounced than we might expect. Think twice before getting online and ordering that "quick fix" diet plan or indulging in a mouthwatering breakfast at your local fast-food restaurant that is guaranteed to stick to your ribs and other places as well!

Chapter 9: Policy. Recognize how policies related to nutrition, health, and exercise are at play in your daily life—in your community, in your state, and in the country as a whole. If you have suggestions or ideas for improving the status quo, don't be afraid to share them with your elected officials. Remember that some policies shift responsibility away from government and place it entirely on our shoulders, which will usually not be effective. What we really need are policies that encourage and support responsible behavior in an environment that promotes health and wellness.

realize when making the changes that will bring about lasting weight loss and improved health. Here are just a few things you can try if you feel you are being overcome by the challenges at hand.

Tap into your social network for support: An advantage of enlisting

Are We There Yet?
How to Define Success

What does success look like where your weight and waistline are concerned? This may seem like an odd question, but it is important if you want to keep the momentum going to change these first few steps into a new approach to a healthy lifestyle. Here are a few tips to keep in mind as you progress in your new, more weight-friendly lifestyle.

"No change" is sometimes a change for the better: For a moment, imagine yourself in a free-falling elevator. We know, it's a terrifying image. Now imagine that the rate of descent starts to slow and soon the elevator has stopped its downward progression. Can you imagine the relief you would feel? The goal of gaining no more weight and hitting stability may be your first stop at success. If you can institute just a few simple changes that achieve this goal and can become healthy habits, you are already on the right track!

Baby steps, believe it or not, are big results: Don't fall into the trap laid by "get thin quick" commercials and weight loss programs. Unrealistic goals can have the negative effect of making you feel that more modest weight loss doesn't matter. On the contrary, science suggests otherwise—modest weight loss is one of the first steps toward a healthier life on so many levels. With this in mind, a goal to lose just 5 percent of your excess weight may be just right for you. If you are successful, congratulations! Try to maintain this for a while, then adjust your goals to gun for another 5 percent or so. The bottom line is that you should feel good about those changes. If you can come away with a greater sense of self-control, you are doing great.

Success is not always about the weight: Even though your weight may have been the motivating factor behind your decision to pick up this book, it is crucial to remember that success is not just measured by weight. Rather, it is better to think of good weight as a symptom that tells you the things you are doing to achieve a healthier lifestyle are working. Remember, you may be able to achieve success in improving the health of your relationships and your quality of life—or perhaps even in your cholesterol levels and blood sugar—before you start to see significant weight change. Consider these benefits, and you may have a tough time saying you are not a success!

your social network rather than just going it alone is the simple fact that you will tap into an existing support system of people who share your desire to change your lifestyle and habits for the better. It's natural at times to feel as if you have little or no control over your weight. But if your approach builds on the strength of other people, your own resolve, too, will be strengthened.

Look for a healthy detour if you are hitting a roadblock: Chances are, if you are looking for a single magic bullet for your weight loss, you will miss your target. Fortunately, throughout the development of your Thinfluence Action Plan, we have given you the tools you need to make changes in any combination of the areas of your life that relate to your weight. This means that if any one particular thing is difficult or impossible to change, you still may be able to improve something else. Say, for example, you can't change the unhealthy aspects of your job or workplace. Why not start at home first? Or if influencing local government policy is too difficult at this time, why not spearhead some healthy initiatives in your own neighborhood, such as a community garden or walking trail?

Do one simple, positive thing. Every day. Without fail: Throughout *Thinfluence*, we have offered an array of tools and strategies—some of which take a great deal of time and effort to implement, but many of which do not. While the approach we have offered is comprehensive in that it deals with many aspects of your life, it is not necessary to change everything at once. Sometimes the best way to get a foothold, especially at the beginning, is to do something simple and make that your new habit. Start with that one simple thing. Perhaps this means instituting a no-sugary-beverage policy in your home—now that's a step that actually saves you the effort of going out to buy something or putting one more thing into your cart. Or perhaps this one simple thing is taking the stairs at work instead of the elevator, or parking further from the entrance. You will find that these small steps are the real building blocks of lasting behavior changes. Make these changes stick, and the healthier weight will follow.

Completing Your Thinfluence Action Plan . . . and Your True Goal

Look back for a minute at the story that started off this chapter. The results of the Team Up 4 Health pilot program, at least for now, appear to have been highly beneficial for most of the participants. A central goal was to build individual and collective resources that would endure, but what happens when the program ends?

This is actually a question that the researchers behind the program wanted to answer. As they followed up with the first-phase participants, they found that most of them maintained the health advancements they had achieved through Team Up 4 Health—achievements such as a better weight, improved blood sugar control, or something else. This program is still ongoing, of course, but these kinds of results after the initial months of the program represent great promise.

For Wilhelmina—who says she wishes she could do the program again—the lasting effects she has enjoyed in her weight and her diet suggest that she incorporated the approaches she learned into her day-to-day life. And she's not keeping quiet about it, either.

"I've already been spreading the word about it," she says with a laugh. "Wherever I go with my brother, I've got a big mouth and I tell everyone about it."

Did Wilhelmina set out to be a positive influence within her community and beyond? Perhaps not at first. But the changes in her lifestyle allowed her to reap the benefits of her new, healthier habits and supportive community, and let her use her own influence to set an example for others.

Now it is time to think about your own goals. Hopefully by now you have compiled a Thinfluence Action Plan that gives you a bounty of options for how you will go about achieving a healthier weight and a healthier lifestyle. You may have already gotten started on these steps and possibly have already seen some results.

So at this point, the goal is to make the best use of your tools to achieve your weight goals and to become a force for positive change in the weight and health of those within your network.

ANALYZE

1. How would you describe where you are in your efforts to achieve or maintain a healthier weight?

   A. In many ways, I am starting my weight loss efforts from square one. Either this is my first real attempt at achieving a healthier weight or the strategies I have tried in the past have not worked for me.

   B. I am currently in the middle of my weight loss journey, and I am looking for additional help in achieving my goals. I feel that I have made at least some progress, but I want to make sure that my gains (or in this case, losses!) can be maintained.

   C. I am at a weight I am happy with. My main motivation for reading this book has been to try and find ways that I can convince others around me to join me in my healthier lifestyle.

2. Which of the choices below best describes your existing infrastructure?

   A. The infrastructure provided by my social circles, my physical environment, and the food and policy environments where I live does not seem supportive of the lifestyle changes that lead to a healthier weight.

   B. While my existing infrastructure is not perfect, I feel that some factors are working in my favor in at least one or two areas—such as a family that stands behind my weight efforts or a favorable food environment where I live.

C. Many elements within my existing infrastructure support my efforts toward a healthier weight—either for myself or for my family and friends.

3. Overall, how challenging do you feel it will be to institute a new plan to achieve or maintain a healthy weight?

   A. While I feel that my goals are attainable, putting my plan into action will likely represent a significant challenge.
   B. I feel that while I am likely to face some hurdles on the way to achieving my weight goals, none of these seem insurmountable.
   C. I feel that it will be relatively easy to institute the necessary changes to my routine, social circles, and outlook toward a healthy lifestyle to make my goals a reality.

ACT

For a moment, look at your answers to the questions. What do your answers look like?

◊ **Mostly As:** It is no secret that you will face some challenging situations in your journey toward a healthier weight. However, using the strategies that have been discussed throughout this book, you will be coming to this fight armed with information that will help you along the way. Remember, every step you take toward creating an environment that supports your efforts at achieving a healthier weight—no matter how small that step is—will bring you closer to the weight you want for yourself.

◊ **Mostly Bs:** Rarely, if ever, are any of us in a slam-dunk situation when we are trying to achieve something meaningful. The good news for you is that a number of factors are likely to work in your favor as you move forward to achieve your weight goals. Better yet, you now have at your disposal the tips and strategies amassed in the course of reading this book. The important thing is to follow through and keep your eyes on your goal.

◊ **Mostly Cs:** It sounds like all of the conditions are right for you to achieve what you want to in terms of your weight or the weight of those close to you. Now it's time to use the strategies you have learned to realize your goals. Good luck!

No matter where you are starting from in your weight loss journey, a few simple approaches may be useful to you going forward:

◊ Start by identifying one behavior of your own that needs to be changed and work to change it. Once you have achieved success in this area, move on to the next challenge in your life.

◊ Create your team and set common goals. Your team should consist of family members, friends, and/or co-workers who will support your efforts and motivate you to achieve a healthier weight.

◊ Add a little taste of competition: See who can walk the most steps at work or who is the most effective at banishing the junk food from the kitchen. Or compete with yourself from week to week in terms of your ability to encourage healthy change. Little contests can go a long way!

◊ Find a mentor, and in turn be a mentor. It is crucial that you find someone who is successful in the domain you seek to better manage in your own life.

INFLUENCE

Now that you have a plan, it is time to share your goals. Get others around you excited about what you are trying to do. Get them involved. Spread your healthy influence in any circle of your life that you can. For you, as well as for those around you, the rewards are clear:

◊ Team spirit; a common goal that will help reinforce the positive actions of all involved

◊ Better health and a more ideal weight through positive lifestyle changes

◊ Stronger relationships within your social network

◊ The feeling of being a force for positive lifestyle change in your family, your workplace, and your community

A Final Word on Thinfluence and What You Have Achieved

So you have reached the final part of the final chapter of *Thinfluence*—and at this point, with any luck, you will be looking at a Thinfluence Action Plan that is full of ideas, tips, and tools you can use to improve your weight and spread your influence.

Is this the end of the road? Far from it; rather, we hope you recognize the plan you have authored over the course of this book as a new beginning—one that helps lead you to not only a healthier weight and healthier lifestyle, but also a certain degree of satisfaction and happiness at having met your goals.

The toolbox you have at your fingertips, the bits of advice you have gleaned and the strategies you have formulated over the course of reading this book—this is all the basis for your very own tailored approach. Realize that these strategies may change as your situation evolves, but the underlying principles you followed to formulate your strategy remain much the same. The key is to understand all of the various influences on your weight and health and to be cognizant of the changes you can make to influence these factors right back.

We hope that by picking up this book, you have attained a greater sense of control over your weight and health destiny, and that of those around you. We hold the keys to changing so many of the aspects of our lives; our weight is one of these. However, we hope it is now apparent that this is in large part an indicator of the healthfulness of our personal relationships and the larger environment in which we live.

Notes

Chapter 1

1   N. A. Christakis and J. H. Fowler, "The Spread of Obesity in a Large Social Network over 32 Years," *New England Journal of Medicine* 357 (2007): 370–9.

2   T. M. Leahey, J. G. LaRose, and J. L. Fava et al., "Social Influences Are Associated with BMI and Weight Loss Intentions in Young Adults," *Obesity* 19 (2011): 1157–62.

3   J. Ludwig, L. Sanbonmatsu, and L. Gennetian et al., "Neighborhoods, Obesity, and Diabetes—A Randomized Social Experiment," *New England Journal of Medicine* 365 (2011): 1509–19.

Chapter 2

1   A. Scuteri, S. Sanna, and W. M. Chen et al., "Genome-Wide Association Scan Shows Genetic Variants in the FTO Gene Are Associated with Obesity-Related Traits," *PLoS Genetics* 3 (2007): e115.

2   T. O. Kilpeläinen, L. Qi, and S. Brage et al., "Physical Activity Attenuates the Influence of FTO Variants on Obesity Risk: A Meta-Analysis of 218,166 Adults and 19,268 Children," *PLoS Medicine* 8 (2011): e1001116.

3   Q. Qi, Y. Li, and A. K. Chomistek et al., "Television Watching, Leisure Time Physical Activity, and the Genetic Predisposition in Relation to Body Mass Index in Women and Men," *Circulation* 126 (2012): 1821–7.

4   Q. Qi, A. Y. Chu, and J. H. Kang et al., "Sugar-Sweetened Beverages and Genetic Risk of Obesity," *New England Journal of Medicine* 367 (2012): 1387–96.

5   D. S. Lauderdale and P. J. Rathouz, "Body Mass Index in a US National Sample of Asian Americans: Effects of Nativity, Years Since Immigration and Socioeconomic Status," *International Journal of Obesity* 24 (2000): 1188–94.

6   R. Oza-Frank and S. A. Cunningham, "The Weight of US Residence among Immigrants: A Systematic Review," *Obesity Reviews* 11 (2010): 271–80.

7   A. Pan, Q. Sun, and S. Czernichow et al., "Bidirectional Association Between Weight Change and Depression in Mid-Aged Women: A Population-Based Longitudinal Study," *International Journal of Obesity* 36 (2012): 595–602.

8   M. Ashwell, P. Gunn, and S. Gibson, "Waist-to-Height Ratio Is a Better Screening Tool Than Waist Circumference and BMI for Adult Cardiometabolic Risk Factors: Systematic Review and Meta-Analysis," *Obesity Reviews* 13 (2011): 275–86.

9   K. A. Scott, S. J. Melhorn, and R. R. Sakai, "Effects of Chronic Social Stress on Obesity," *Current Obesity Reports* 1 (2012): 16–25.

10   A. J. Stunkard and S. Messick, "The Three-Factor Eating Questionnaire to Measure Dietary Restraint, Disinhibition and Hunger," *Journal of Psychosomatic Research* 29 (1985): 71–83.

11   A. N. Gearhardt, C. M. Grilo, and R. J. DiLeone et al., "Can Food Be Addictive? Public Health and Policy Implications," *Addiction* 106 (2011): 1208–12.

12   B. S. Lennerz, D. C. Alsop, and L. M. Holsen et al., "Effects of Dietary Glycemic Index on Brain Regions Related to Reward and Craving in Men," *American Journal of Clinical Nutrition* 98 (2013): 641–7.

13   A. N. Gearhardt, W. R. Corbin, and K. D. Brownell, "Preliminary Validation of the Yale Food Addiction Scale," *Appetite* 52 (2009): 430–6.

14   S. M. Mason, A. J. Flint, and A. E. Field et al.,"Abuse Victimization in Childhood or Adolescence and Risk of Food Addiction in Adult Women," *Obesity* 21 (2013): E7775–81.

15   N. D. Volkow, G. Wang, and R. D. Baler, "Reward, Dopamine and the Control of Food Intake: Implications for Obesity," *Trends in Cognitive Sciences* 15 (2011): 37–46.

16   K. D. Brownell, R. Kersh, and D. S. Ludwig et al., "Personal Responsibility and Obesity: A Constructive Approach to a Controversial Issue," *Health Affairs* 29 (2010): 379–87.

Chapter 3

1   NPR, Robert Wood Johnson Foundation, and Harvard School of Public Health, "A Poll about Children and Weight," www.rwjf.org/en/research-publications/find-rwjf-research/2013/02/a-poll-about-children-and-weight.html (2013).

2   K. Van Ittersum and B. Wansink, "Plate Size and Color Suggestibility: The Delboeuf Illusion's Bias on Serving and Eating Behavior," *Journal of Consumer Research* 39 (2012): 215–28.

3   K. I. DiSantis, L. L. Birch, and A. Davey et al., "Plate Size and Children's Appetite: Effects of Larger Dishware on Self-Served Portions and Intake," *Pediatrics* 131 (2013): e1451–8.

4   A. Drewnowski and Nicole Darmon, "The Economics of Obesity: Dietary Energy Density and Energy Cost," *American Journal of Clinical Nutrition* 82 (2005): 265S–73S.

5   T. Østbye, R. L. Kolotkin, and H. He et al., "Sexual Functioning in Obese Adults Enrolling in a Weight Loss Study," *Journal of Sex & Marital Therapy* 37 (2011): 224–35.

6   S. P. Efstathiou, I. I. Skeva, and E. Zorbala et al., "Metabolic Syndrome in Adolescence: Can It Be Predicted from Natal and Parental Profile? The Prediction of Metabolic Syndrome in Adolescence (PREMA) Study," *Circulation* 125 (2012): 902–10.

7   K. Preiss, L. Brennan, and D. Clarke, "A Systematic Review of Variables Associated with the Relationship between Obesity and Depression," *Obesity Reviews* 14 (2013): 906–18.

8   C. Dong, L. E. Sanchez, and R. A. Price, "Relationship of Obesity to Depression: A Family-Based Study," *International Journal of Obesity and Related Metabolic Disorders* 28 (2004): 790–5.

9   F. Koch, A. Sepa, and J. Ludvigsson, "Psychological Stress and Obesity," *Journal of Pediatrics* 153 (2008): 839–44.

10   A. Sanchez-Villegas, A. E. Field, and E. J. O'Reilly et al., "Perceived and Actual Obesity in Childhood and Adolescence and Risk of Adult Depression," *Journal of Epidemiology and Public Health* 67 (2013): 81–86.

Chapter 4

1   L. F. Berkman and S. L. Syme, "Social Networks, Host Resistance, and Mortality: A Nine-Year Follow-Up Study of Alameda County Residents," *American Journal of Epidemiology* 109 (1979): 186–204.

2   I. Kawachi, G. A. Colditz, and A. Ascherio et al., "A Prospective Study of Social Networks in Relation to Total Mortality and Cardiovascular Disease in Men in the USA," *Journal of Epidemiology and Community Health* 50 (1996): 245–51.

3   C. Segrin and S. A. Passalacqua, "Functions of Loneliness, Social Support, Health Behaviors, and Stress in Association with Poor Health," *Health Communication* 25 (2010): 312–22.

4   C. J. Packard, J. Cavanagh, and J. S. McLean et al., "Interaction of Personality Traits with Social Deprivation in Determining Mental Wellbeing and Health Behaviours," *Journal of Public Health* 34 (2012): 615–24.

5   S. L. Tamers, C. Okechukwu, and J. Allen et al., "Are Social Relationships a Healthy Influence on Obesogenic Behaviors among Racially/Ethnically Diverse and Socio-Economically Disadvantaged Residents?" *Preventive Medicine* 56 (2013): 70–74.

6   R. C. J. Hermans, A. Lichtwarck-Aschoff, and K. E. Bevelander et al., "Mimicry of Food Intake: The Dynamic Interplay between Eating Companions," *PLoS ONE* 7 (2012) e31027.

7   J. J. Exline, A. L. Zell, and E. Bratslavsky et al., "People-Pleasing through Eating: Sociotropy Predicts Greater Eating in Response to Perceived Social Pressure," *Journal of Social and Clinical Psychology* 31 (2012): 169–93.

8   Y. Zhang, X. Li, and T. Wang, "Identifying Influencers in Online Social Networks: The Role of Tie Strength," *International Journal of Intelligent Information Technologies* 9 (2013): 1–20.

9   S. D. Young, L. Harrell, and D. Jaganath et al., "Feasibility of Recruiting Peer Educators for an Online Social Networking-Based Health Intervention," *Health Education Journal* 72 (2013): 276–82.

10   D. B. Bahr, R. C. Browning, and H. R. Wyatt et al., "Exploiting Social Networks to Mitigate the Obesity Epidemic," *Obesity* 17 (2009): 723–8.

11   S. Heshka, J. W. Anderson, and R. L. Atkinson et al., "Weight Loss with Self-Help Compared with a Structured Commercial Program," *JAMA* 289 (2003): 1792–8.

12   M. L. Dansinger, J. A. Gleason, and J. L. Griffith et al., "Comparison of the Atkins, Ornish, Weight Watchers, and Zone Diets for Weight Loss and Heart Disease Risk Reduction," *JAMA* 293 (2005): 43–53.

13   C. A. Johnston, S. Rost, and K. Miller-Kovach et al., "A Randomized Controlled Trial of a Community-based Behavioral Counseling Program," *American Journal of Medicine* 126 (2013): 1143.e19-24.

14   A. L. Ahern, A. D. Olson, and L. M. Aston et al., "Weight Watchers on Prescription: An Observational Study of Weight Change among Adults Referred to Weight Watchers by the NHS," *BMC Public Health* 11 (2011): 434.

15   A. L. Ahern, A. D. Olsen, and L. M. Aston, "An Audit of the UK Weight Watchers NHS Referral Scheme," *Obesity Facts* (2010).

Chapter 5

1   L. Quintiliani, J. Sattelmair, and G. Sorensen, "The Workplace as a Setting for Interventions to Improve Diet and Promote Physical Activity: Background Paper Prepared for the WHO/WEF Joint Event on Preventing Noncommunicable Diseases in the Workplace," Dalian/China (2007).

2   J. N. Morris, J. A. Heady, and P. A. B. Raffle et al., "Coronary Heart-Disease and Physical Activity of Work," *Lancet* 262 (1953): 1111–20.

3   J. A. Levine, L. M. Lanningham-Foster, and S. K. McCrady et al., "Interindividual Variation in Posture Allocation: Possible Role in Human Obesity," *Science* 307 (2005): 584–6.

4   J. A. Levine, S. J. Schleusner, and M. D. Jensen, "Energy Expenditure of Nonexercise Activity," *American Journal of Clinical Nutrition* 72 (2000): 1451–4.

5   L. Lanningham-Foster, L. J. Nysse, and J. A. Levine, "Labor Saved, Calories Lost: The Energetic Impact of Domestic Labor-Saving Devices," *Obesity Research* 11, (2003): 1178–81.

6   S. K. McCrady and J. A. Levine, "Sedentariness at Work: How Much Do We Really Sit?" *Obesity* 17 (2009): 2103–5.

7   A. Pan, E. S. Schernhammer, and Q. Sun et al., "Rotating Night Shift Work and Risk of Type 2 Diabetes: Two Prospective Cohort Studies in Women," *PLoS Medicine* 8 (2011): e1001141.

8   D. W. Byrne, R. Z. Goetzel, and P. W. McGown et al., "Seven-Year Trends in Employee Health Habits from a Comprehensive Workplace Health Promotion Program at Vanderbilt University," *Journal of Occupational and Environmental Medicine* 53 (2011): 1372–81.

9   A. N. Thorndike, L. Sonnenberg, and J. Riis et al., "A 2-Phase Labeling and Choice Architecture Intervention to Improve Healthy Food and Beverage Choices," *American Journal of Public Health* 102 (2012): 584.

Chapter 6

1   R. A. Dunn, "The Effect of Fast-Food Availability on Obesity: An Analysis by Gender, Race, and Residential Location," *American Journal of Agricultural Economics* 92 (2010): 1149–64.

2   K. B. Morland and K. R. Evenson, "Obesity Prevalence and the Local Food Environment," *Health & Place* 15 (2009): 491–5.

3   F. Li, P. Harmer, and B. J. Cardinal et al., "Obesity and the Built Environment: Does the Density of Neighborhood Fast-Food Outlets Matter?" *American Journal of Health Promotion* 23 (2009): 203–9.

4   A. M. Bernstein, D. E. Bloom, and B. A. Rosner et al., "Relation of Food Cost to Healthfulness of Diet among US Women," *American Journal of Clinical Nutrition* 92 (2010): 1197–1203.

5   D. Mozaffarian, T. Hao, and E. B. Rimm et al., "Changes in Diet and Lifestyle and Long-Term Weight Gain in Women and Men," *New England Journal of Medicine* 364 (2011): 2392–404.

6   D. M. Gibson, "The Neighborhood Food Environment and Adult Weight Status: Estimates from Longitudinal Data," *American Journal of Public Health* 101 (2011): 71–8.

7   D. B. Reed, P. J. Patterson, and N. Wasserman, "Obesity in Rural Youth: Looking Beyond Nutrition and Physical Activity," *Journal of Nutrition Education and Behavior* 43 (2011): 401–8.

8   C. Gordon, M. Purciel-Hill, and N. R. Ghai et al., "Measuring Food Deserts in New York City's Low-Income Neighborhoods," *Health & Place* 17 (2011): 696–700.

9   A. Singh, L. Uijtdewilligen, and J. W. R. Twisk et al., "Physical Activity and Performance at School: A Systematic Review of the Literature Including a Methodological Quality Assessment," *Archives of Pediatrics & Adolescent Medicine* 166 (2012): 49.

Chapter 7

1   E. Robinson, P. Aveyard, and A. Daley et al., "Eating Attentively: A Systematic Review and Meta-Analysis of the Effect of Food Intake Memory and Awareness on Eating," *American Journal of Clinical Nutrition* 97 (2013): 728–42.

2   E. van Kleef, M. Shimizu, and B. Wansink, "Serving Bowl Selection Biases the Amount of Food Served," *Journal of Nutrition Education and Behavior* 44 (2012): 66–70.

3   B. Wansink, "Measuring Food Intake in Field Studies," *Handbook of Assessment Methods for Eating Behaviors and Weight-Related Problems: Measures, Theory, and Research* (2009): 327.

4   D. Walker, L. Smarandescu, and B. Wansink, "Half Full or Empty: Cues That Lead Wine Drinkers to Unintentionally Overpour," *Substance Use & Misuse* (2013).

5   J. A. Steeves, D. L. Thompson, and D. R. Bassett Jr., "Energy Cost of Stepping in Place While Watching Television Commercials," *Medicine and Science in Sports and Exercise* 44 (2012): 330–5.

6   Go Sox.

7   K. R. Smith, B. B. Brown, and I. Yamada et al., "Walkability and Body Mass Index: Density, Design, and New Diversity Measures," *American Journal of Preventive Medicine* 35 (2008): 237–44.

8   T. S. Church, D. M. Thomas, and C. Tudor-Locke et al., "Trends over 5 Decades in US Occupation-Related Physical Activity and Their Associations with Obesity," *PloS ONE* 6 (2011): e19657.

9   J. A. Steeves, D. R. Bassett, and D. L. Thompson et al., "Relationships of Occupational and Non-Occupational Physical Activity to Abdominal Obesity," *International Journal of Obesity* 36 (2011): 100–6.

10   Curious as to how your own area stacks up? You can visit the Bike Score site (www.walkscore.com/bike) to find out.

Chapter 8

1   A. Grøntved and F. B. Hu, "Television Viewing and Risk of Type 2 Diabetes, Cardiovascular Disease, and All-Cause Mortality," *JAMA* 305 (2011): 2448.

2   F. J. Zimmerman and J. F. Bell, "Associations of Television Content Type and Obesity in Children," *American Journal of Public Health* 100 (2010): 334–40.

3   M. Scully, H. Dixon, and M. Wakefield, "Association between Commercial Television Exposure and Fast-Food Consumption among Adults," *Public Health Nutrition* 12 (2009): 105–10.

4   V. C. Strasburger, A. B. Jordan, and E. Donnerstein, "Health Effects of Media on Children and Adolescents," *Pediatrics* 125 (2010): 756–67.

5   W. Gantz, N. Schwartz, and J. R. Angelini et al., "Food for Thought: Television Food Advertising to Children in the United States," a Henry J. Kaiser Family Foundation report (2007).

6   J. Cawley, R. Avery, and M. Eisenberg, "The Effect of Advertising and Deceptive Advertising on Consumption: The Case of Over-the-Counter Weight Loss Products," Working Paper, www. iza.org/conference_files/riskonomics2011/cawley_j6697.pdf (2011).

7   P. L. Ching, W. C. Willett, and E. B. Rimm et al., "Activity Level and Risk of Overweight in Male Health Professionals," *American Journal of Public Health* 86 (1996): 25–30.

8   F. B. Hu, T. Y. Li, and G. A. Colditz et al., "Television Watching and Other Sedentary Behaviors in Relation to Risk of Obesity and Type 2 Diabetes Mellitus in Women," *JAMA* 289 (2003): 1785–91.

9   L. M. Powell, J. L. Harris, and T. Fox, "Food Marketing Expenditures Aimed at Youth: Putting the Numbers in Context," *American Journal of Preventive Medicine* 45 (2013): 453–61.

10   B. B. Duncan, L. E. Chambless, and M. I. Schmidt et al., "Association of the Waist-to-Hip Ratio Is Different with Wine Than with Beer or Hard Liquor Consumption," *American Journal of Epidemiology* 142 (1995): 1034–8.

11   A. L. Franks, S. H. Kelder, and G. A. Dino et al., "Peer Reviewed: School-Based Programs: Lessons Learned from CATCH, Planet Health, and Not-On-Tobacco," *Preventing Chronic Disease* 4 (2007): A33.

12   J. L. Harris, M. B. Schwartz, and K. D. Brownell et al., "Fast Food FACTS: Evaluating Fast Food Nutrition and Marketing to Youth. 2010," *Rudd Center for Food Policy and Obesity* (2012).

13   K. Weber, M. Story, and L. Harnack, "Internet Food Marketing Strategies Aimed at Children and Adolescents: A Content Analysis of Food and Beverage Brand Web Sites," *Journal of the American Dietetic Association* 106 (2006) 1463–6.

Chapter 9

1   S. C. Kulkarni, A. Levin-Rector, and M. Ezzati et al., "Falling Behind: Life Expectancy in US Counties from 2000 to 2007 in an International Context," *Population Health Metrics* 9 (2011): 16.

2   Gallup-Healthways Well-Being Index (2012), www.healthways.com/solution/default.aspx?id=1125.

3   B. A. Swinburn, G. Sacks, K. D. Hall, K. McPherson, D. T. Finegood, M. L. Moodie, and S. L. Gortmaker, "The Global Obesity Pandemic: Shaped by Global Drivers and Local Environments," *Lancet* 378 (2011): 801–14.

4   K. D. Brownell, R. Kersh, and D. S. Ludwig et al., "Personal Responsibility and Obesity: A Constructive Approach to a Controversial Issue," *Health Affairs* 29 (2010): 379–87.

5   C. W. Leung, W. C. Willett, and E. L. Ding, "Low-Income Supplemental Nutrition Assistance Program Participation Is Related to Adiposity and Metabolic Risk Factors," *American Journal of Clinical Nutrition* 95 (2012): 17–24.

6   J. D. Shenkin and M. F. Jacobson, "Using the Food Stamp Program and Other Methods to Promote Healthy Diets for Low-Income Consumers," *American Journal of Public Health* 100 (2010): 1562–4.

7   C. W. Leung, E. L. Ding, and P. J. Catalano et al., "Dietary Intake and Dietary Quality of Low-Income Adults in the Supplemental Nutrition Assistance Program," *American Journal of Clinical Nutrition* 96 (2012): 977–88.

8   B. Wansink and K. Van Ittersum, "Shape of Glass and Amount of Alcohol Poured: Comparative Study of Effect of Practice and Concentration," *BMJ* 331 (2005): 1512.

9   J. Sobal and B. Wansink, "Kitchenscapes, Tablescapes, Platescapes, and Foodscapes: Influences of Microscale Built Environments on Food Intake," *Environment and Behavior* 39 (2007): 124–42.

10   A. L. Cradock, A. McHugh, and H. Mont-Ferguson et al., "Effect of School District Policy Change on Consumption of Sugar-Sweetened Beverages among High School Students, Boston, Massachusetts, 2004-2006," *Preventing Chronic Disease* 8 (2011): A74.

11   K. H. K. Yeary, C. E. Cornell, and P. Moore, "Peer Reviewed: Feasibility of an Evidence-Based Weight Loss Intervention for a Faith-Based, Rural, African American Population," *Preventing Chronic Disease* 8 (2011): A146.

12   A. J. McMichael, J. W. Powles, and C. D. Butler et al., "Food, Livestock Production, Energy, Climate Change, and Health," *Lancet* 370 (2007): 1253–63.

13   E. A. Finkelstein, J. G. Trogdon, and J. W. Cohen et al., "Annual Medical Spending Attributable to Obesity: Payer- and Service-Specific Estimates," *Health Affairs* 28 (2009): w822–31.

14   J. Cawley and C. Meyerhoefer, "The Medical Care Costs of Obesity: An Instrumental Variables Approach," *Journal of Health Economics* 31 (2012): 219–30.

15   C. Mitchell, G. Cowburn, and C. Foster, "Assessing the Options for Local Government to Use Legal Approaches to Combat Obesity in the UK: Putting Theory into Practice," *Obesity Reviews* 12 (2011): 660–7.

16   J. L. Harris and S. K. Graff, "Protecting Children from Harmful Food Marketing: Options for Local Government to Make a Difference," *Preventing Chronic Disease* 8 (2011) A92.

Acknowledgments

As with most projects that are worth undertaking, there are a long list of people and institutions without whose contributions *Thinfluence* would not have been possible. Special thanks goes to Chief Editor of Books at Harvard Health Publications Julie Silver, MD, who assembled our team and provided much of the momentum that allowed us to turn our findings and observations into this book. We are likewise indebted to the rest of the team at Harvard Health Publications. Our gratitude extends as well to our literary agent Linda Konner for her guidance and support throughout this effort.

We would also like to thank Rodale for seeing the potential in this project, as well as to Ursula Cary and Trisha Calvo for their editorial guidance.

Walter Willett and Malissa Wood would like to acknowledge their colleagues at Harvard and its affiliated institutions who are advancing the research discussed in this work, particularly those whose research and expertise have been cited in this work. Walter would additionally like to acknowledge the participants in the Nurses' Health Studies and Health Professional's Follow-up Study, who have shared their experiences for the last four decades, which has taught us much of what we now know about diet and health. Malissa would also like to thank her patients, many of whom have struggled with and overcome health obstacles, including obesity. For her, working with these patients has been a source of wisdom and experience every day, particularly when it comes to helping others in their situations. Dan Childs would like to thank his colleagues at ABC News for their support of this effort.

Last, but certainly not least, we would like to express our gratitude to those who shared the personal stories that have been featured in several chapters of this book. It is our hope that your experiences will help inspire and influence others in their own efforts to improve their weight and their lives.

Index

Boldface page references indicate illustrations. Underscored references indicate boxed text.

workplace, 112
of yourself on others, 8–9, 11–12
Infrastructure, 214–15
Inheritance. *See* Family; Genetics
Inner-self factors. *See also* Personal responsibility
  common traits blamed for weight, 21
  emotions, 28–34
  external factors affecting, 22, 23–24, 37–38
  food addiction, 34–37
  genetics, 24–28
  impact on weight, 22–24
  recap of important messages, <u>218</u>
  Thinfluence Action Plan for, 38–41
iPhone, as weight-control tool, <u>146–47</u>

J

Jacobson, Michael, <u>190</u>, <u>191</u>
Japan, obesity rate in, 27–28
Japan, weight ranking of, <u>187</u>

K

Kaiser Family Foundation, 163, 164
Katzen, Mollie, 133, xi
Kawachi, Ichiro, 71

L

Late-shift work, diabetes risk due to, 102
Laurie M. Tisch Illumination Fund, <u>201</u>
Learn to Be Lean program, 68–69, 73
Leung, Cindy, <u>191</u>
Levine, James, 99, <u>100</u>
Lifestyle. *See also* Physical activity
  genetic risk of obesity triggered by, 26–27
  support groups for, 78–82
Ludwig, David, 34

M

Magic bullet approaches, 166–71, 221
Makarechi, Leila, 213
Marketing. *See* Advertising and marketing
Massachusetts General Hospital (MGH)
  Be Fit program at, 95–96, 106, 113
  Cardiovascular Disease Prevention Center at, 68
  HAPPY Heart Study at, 73, 80–81, xii
MCI, 210–11
Media. *See also* Advertising and marketing; Social media; TV
  children's consumption of, 163
  in Circles of Influence, 176
  educating children about, <u>173</u>
  food porn, <u>168–69</u>
  genetics misinformation in, 25–26
  health news headlines, <u>172</u>
  limiting exposure to, 179
  messages about weight in, x
  online, 171, 172, <u>174–75</u>, 180

promoting community ideas via, 206
  public service announcements, 164–65
  recap of important messages, <u>219</u>
  Thinfluence Action Plan, 177–81
  unhealthy messages in, 166–68
Mediterranean diet, <u>19</u>
Mentors and mentoring, 225
Meyerhoefer, Chad, <u>199</u>
Microclinic International (MCI), 210–11
Mindless Eating, <u>142</u>
Motivation, 70, 71–72. *See also* Influence

N

National Health and Nutrition Examination Survey, <u>149</u>
Neighborhood "bikeability," <u>150–51</u>
Neighborhood food environment, 124–26
Netherlands, weight ranking of, <u>187</u>
New York City policies, <u>192</u>, 199, <u>200–201</u>
No eating zones at home, <u>157</u>
NPR, 49
Nudge factor, <u>86</u>
Nurses' Health Study, 28–30, 36, xi
Nurses' Health Study II, 36
Nurturer archetype, 48–50
Nutritionists, help from, 60–61

O

Obesity and overweight
  in Bell County, Kentucky, 210
  costs to society, <u>198–99</u>
  deaths from smoking vs., <u>192</u>
  depression linked to, 28–30
  epidemic of, 5
  fast food availability increasing risk of, <u>118</u>
  genetics' influence on, 24–27
  "go it alone" attitude toward, 5, ix–x
  in Holmes County, Mississippi, 183
  personal responsibility framing approaches to, 38, 187–88
  poverty linked to, <u>190</u>
  SNAP participation and, <u>190–91</u>
  social contagion for, 4
  social network's affect on, 71
  US rate of, <u>187</u>
Office culture, 100–101, 106–7. *See also* Work environment
Oliver, Jamie, <u>128</u>
O'Neill, Tip, <u>198</u>
Online media, 171, 172, <u>174–75</u>, 180. *See also* Social media
Organized groups. *See* Support groups
Overweight. *See* Obesity and overweight

P

Palatable snacking, 30–31
Pan, An, 30